FIRST AID
Step by Step

John Camm and Tim McCarthy

Illustrated by David Eaton

AF526883

CBS

CBS PUBLISHERS & DISTRIBUTORS PVT. LTD.

New Delhi • Bangalore • Pune • Cochin • Chennai (India)

ISBN : 81-239-0993-4

First Indian Reprint : 1991
Reprint : 2002, 2003

Copyright © John Camm & Tim McCarthy

This edition has been reprinted in India by arrangement with Heinemann Professional Publishing Limited, London

All rights reserved. No part of this book may be reproduced or transmitted in any form or by any means, electronic or mechanical, including photocopying, recording, or any information storage and retrieval system without permission, in writing, from the publisher.

Sales Territory : India only

Published by Satish Kumar Jain and produced by V.K. Jain for
CBS Publishers & Distributors Pvt. Ltd.,
CBS Plaza, 4819/XI Prahlad Street, 24 Ansari Road, Daryaganj,
New Delhi - 110002, India. • Website: www.cbspd.com
e-mail: delhi@cbspd.com, cbspubs@airtelmail.in
Ph.: 23289259, 23266861, 23266867 • Fax: 011-23243014

Branches:

- ***Bengaluru:*** Seema House, 2975, 17th Cross, K.R. Road, Bansankari 2nd Stage, Bengaluru - 560070
  • Ph.: +91-80-26771678/79 • Fax: +91-80-26771680
  • E-mail: cbsbng@gmail.com, bangalore@cbspd.com
- ***Pune:*** Bhuruk Prestige, Sr. No. 52/12/2+1+3/2, Narhe, Haveli (Near Katraj-Dehu Road By-pass), Pune - 411041
  • Ph.: +91-20-64704058/59, 32342277 • E-mail: pune@cbspd.com
- ***Kochi:*** 36/14, Kalluvilakam, Lissie Hospital Road, Kochi - 682018, Kerala • Ph.: +91-484-4059061-65
  • Fax: +91-484-4059065 • E-mail: cochin@cbspd.com
- ***Chennai:*** 20, West Park Road, Shenoy Nagar, Chennai - 600030
  Ph.: +91-44-26260666, 26208620 • Fax: +91-44-42032115
  • E-mail: chennai@cbspd.com

Printed at :
Neekunj Print Process, Delhi

Contents

To Young First-Aiders, especially our own pupils at Gravesend

Introduction

When an accident occurs, the first impulse of most young people is to help the victim, yet few have sufficient knowledge to achieve this goal. First aid is the skill of applying common sense in such a way that suffering ends, life is saved and recovery begins. Although it is a complex subject the two most important things to know are how to:

stop the victim bleeding
and
keep him breathing

until professional help arrives. This is the first principle of all first aid and the basis on which *First Aid Step by Step* is written.

The book will acquaint young readers with emergency situations that may require first aid and give the remedies necessary to deal with them in simple step by step fashion. Each chapter begins with a hypothetica problem, is followed by a theory section which discusses the biologica and medical aspects and an illustrated guide on how to cope with the victim's injury, and finishes with a short quiz.

Much of the mechanical detail about fractures, bandages and transport which normally clutters first aid books has been taken out o the main part and put into the Appendices at the back. The result is a book which conveys complex information in a simple way and is easy to use.

Test your first-aid knowledge. As you begin a new chapter, read the problem on the first page and then on a separate piece of paper write down your method of dealing with the situation. When you finish the chapter check your paper and do the short quiz.

1 Is it a poison?

You go into your friend's house and find his young brother lying on the floor. He is very drowsy, has a bluish colour and his breathing is shallow. You listen to his chest and hear his heart beating rapidly. Close by is a bottle containing a few of his mother's pills. Thinking they were sweets, he ate some and has poisoned himself.

What would you do to save his life?

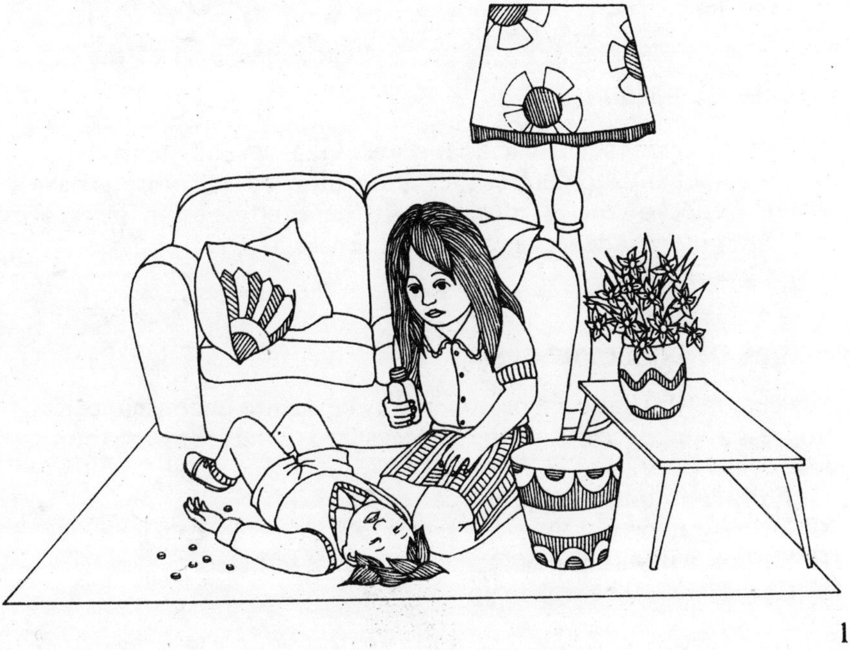

Theory

A poison is a substance which is harmful to the body. If too much of almost anything is taken it may be poisonous.
Poisons include:
Gases such as coal gas (containing carbon monoxide), sulphur dioxide, etc.
Tablets such as heart or nerve pills
Liquids such as weedkillers, bleaches and acids
Plants such as toadstools, laburnum, etc.

Usually taken into the mouth, poisons pass through the gullet or oesophagus and into the stomach. Two tubes pass downwards from the back of the mouth; the one at the front is the windpipe or trachea; at the back is the gullet. The stomach is a bag-like enlargement of the gut which acts like a reservoir for food. Digestion starts here.

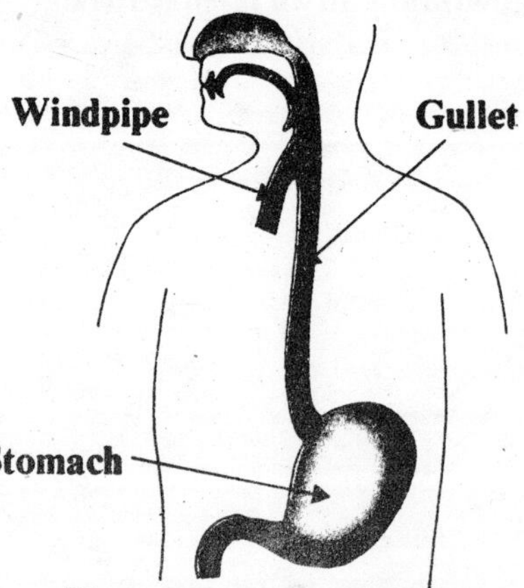

The upper part of the gut

Effects of poison

Corrosive poisons such as acids and weedkillers usually burn the mouth, gullet and stomach as they are swallowed. All poisons have a powerful effect on the nervous system either exciting (as in the case of amphetamines) or depressing it (as in the case of barbiturates or sleeping tablets).

Stages of consciousness

Any person who has been poisoned may lapse into unconsciousness. Progress of unconscious victims is measured in the following four stages:

I Fully conscious: awake and can talk sensibly
II Drowsy: awake at times but seems to dose off. Speech is slurred
III Stupor: will wake up only if severe pain is inflicted
IV Coma: cannot be woken up

How can I help ?

The First Aider has a special opportunity in the case of poisons as only swift action will save the life of the victim.
If the victim is conscious, is breathing without difficulty and has a satisfactory pulse, check whether the poison has caused any corrosion. This will be indicated by burns in or around the mouth. (see opposite)

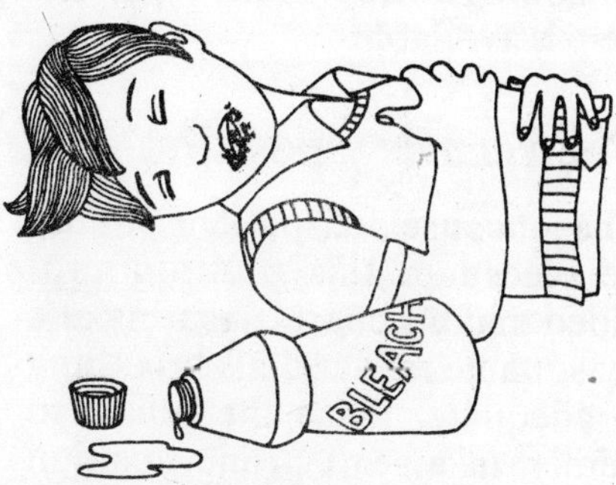

Provided that there is no corrosion, induce vomiting by:

—forcing two fingers down the victim's throat

OR

—making him drink a mixture of salt and water

OR

—a solution of mustard and water

OR

—Ipecac syrup

If the victim's mouth is burnt dilute the poison with water or milk to neutralize its corrosive effects. Treat any pain caused by the corrosion with something soothing such as ice cream or olive oil. Do *not* make the victim vomit as this will only result in the same corrosive poison burning the mouth and gullet again. It could even burn through the gullet wall and this would be a very serious complication.
Both corrosive and non-corrosive poisons may be treated with activated charcoal. This substance consists of fine, specially prepared charcoal particles which are mixed with water and swallowed. This prevents the absorption of a wide variety of poisonous substances.

Intentional overdose

Self-poisoning is an important and not uncommon cause of serious illness and even death. The poisonous substances used are usually sleeping tablets or pain-killing medicines. Gas poisoning is now rare but intentional poisoning with garden and domestic agents is increasing. Although there are two possible motives for taking an overdose,—a genuine wish to die or a rather desperate way of asking for help,—it must always be assumed that the victim seriously intended to kill himself. First aid care should involve treatment of the poisoning and constant supervision of the victim until expert medical help is available.

The recovery position

The unconscious patient should be placed in this position provided that his heart is beating at a reasonable rate and his breathing is adequate. Place the poisoned person in a semi prone position with his head down. This will ensure that the tongue falls forward leaving the airways open. If the victim is sick, the vomit will come out of the mouth and not choke the lungs.

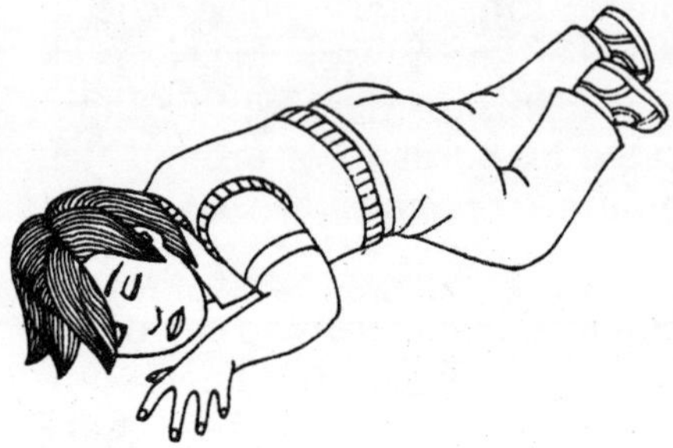

Drug addiction

Addiction to dangerous drugs is a growing problem among young people and school children. No-one can experiment with these drugs without running the risk of being permanently trapped. The common addictive drugs can be divided into three types. (See opposite)

The addict may be recognised by his strange behaviour and sometimes by needle-marks and skin infections where drugs have been injected. Drug addiction can kill, or ruin the lives of both the addict and his family. The best cure is prevention but if a person is already 'hooked' on drugs, early treatment may help him overcome his addiction. Persuade any addict you know to see his doctor.—Do not allow him to keep his awful secret—it could kill him!

Effects of alcohol

Small quantities of alcohol can produce a pleasant state of mind,—large quantities dull the brain, impair breathing and may eventually cause death. The drunk is in danger in several ways: he may have an accident, be sick and fill his lungs with vomit, or develop cold exhaustion. Keep him warm and stop him injuring himself. If he is paralytic place him in the recovery position and get medical help.

Type	Proper Name	Drug Slang	Effects
Stimulants	Amphetamines	Bennies, purple hearts, dex etc.	These drugs produce excitement and over-activity. At times the addict is over-aggressive and cannot sleep.
	Cocaine	coke, snow etc.	
Depressants	Barbiturates	Sleepers, blues, barbs etc.	Drugs such as these dull the mind and slow the person down.
	Heroin	Gunk, 'H' etc.	Although they feel physically well, their mental performance is poor.
Mind Expanders	Cannabis	Pot, hash, grass etc.	These drugs give rise to vivid images, nightmares and dreamlike states.
	L.S.D.	Acid, strawberry fields.	

Step by Step

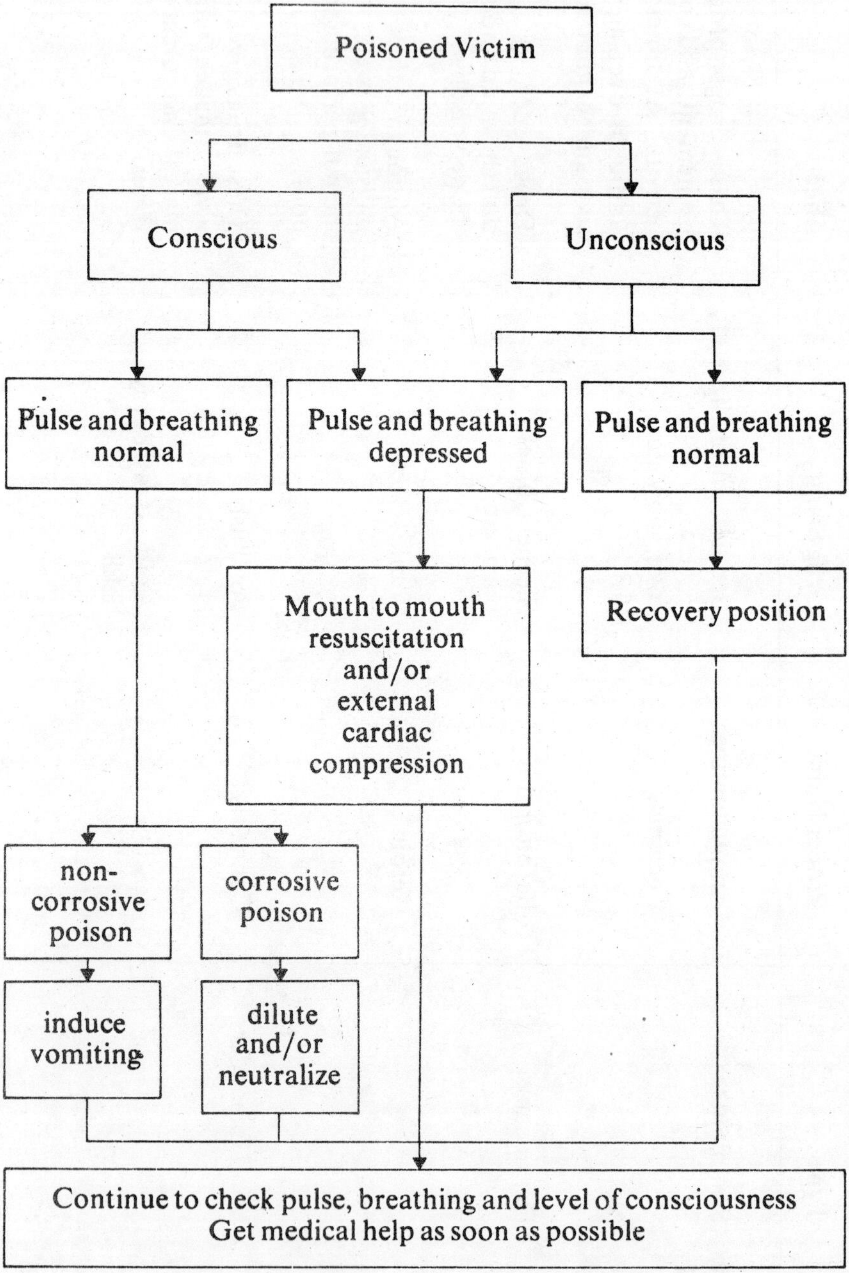
Poisoned Victim
Conscious
Unconscious
Pulse and breathing normal
Pulse and breathing depressed
Pulse and breathing normal
Mouth to mouth resuscitation and/or external cardiac compression
Recovery position
non-corrosive poison
corrosive poison
induce vomiting
dilute and/or neutralize
Continue to check pulse, breathing and level of consciousness
Get medical help as soon as possible

Do's	Dont's
Check level of consciousness, pulse and breathing regularly and record your results	Do *not* give an unconscious victim anything to drink
Look for evidence of the type of poison taken and see if any note of explanation has been left by the victim	Do *not* make an unconscious victim vomit
Get medical help as soon as possible	Do *not* induce vomiting if the poison is corrosive

Gas poisoning

The commonest poisonous gas in the home is carbon monoxide. This is present in coal gas but not in North Sea or natural gas. It is also found in exhausts from petrol engines. The victim of carbon monoxide poisoning will be cherry red in colour and will breathe with difficulty. The colour is caused by the carbon monoxide combining with the blood pigment haemoglobin.

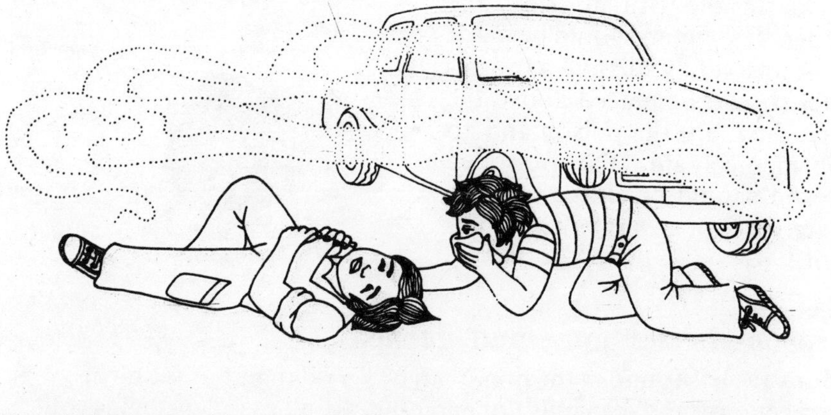

You should get to the victim without gassing yourself. Put a cloth over your mouth and quickly approach the victim. Immediately pull the victim into fresh air and start mouth to mouth resuscitation if the victim is either fighting for his breath or has stopped breathing. Check pulse and state of consciousness regularly.

Wasp and bee stings

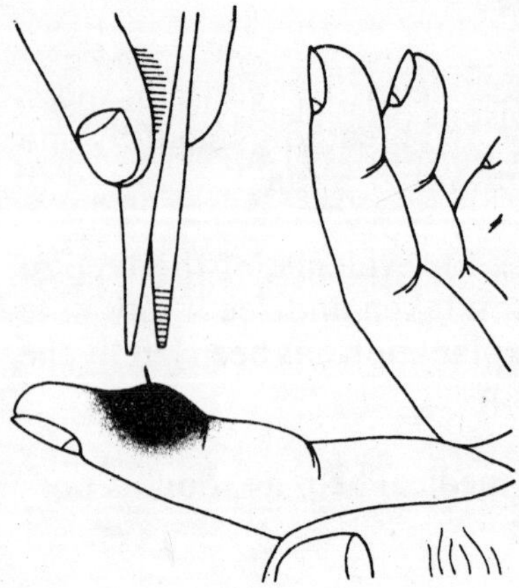

Remove the sting from the bite with a pair of tweezers. Rinse the wound with a solution of bicarbonate of soda. A soothing lotion such as calamine can be applied. If there is much swelling apply an ice pack. Stings inside the mouth may be dangerous as swelling can interfere with breathing. In this case wash the mouth out with sodium bicarbonate and suck on ice.

Dog, rodent and human bites

Treat as simple dirty wounds (see chapter 8)

Jelly Fish

These animals produce itchy nettle-rash like stings and can be treated with calamine lotion.

Snake bites

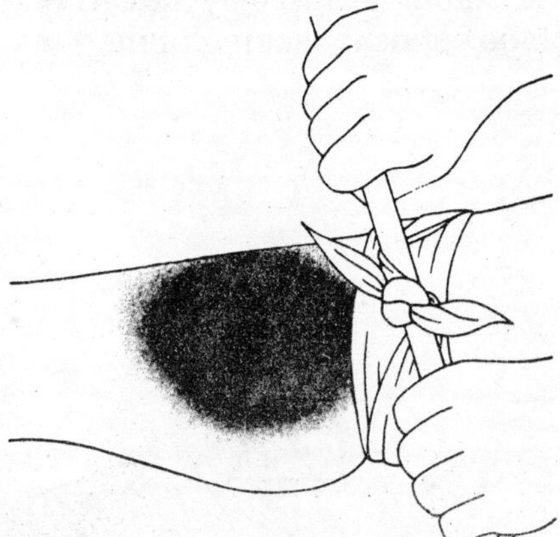

There is only one poisonous snake in the British Isles—the adder. The victim should be made to lie absolutely still and a tourniquet should be placed above the bite. Suck out the poison and go for medical aid. The poisoned person should on *no* account be given alcohol or any other stimulant.

Poisons in the home and garden

Many tablets found in the home can be very dangerous. Aspirins, paracetamol and iron pills, for example, are all useful medicines but can be poisonous if too many are taken. Coloured tablets are often mistaken for sweets and eaten by unsuspecting children. Keep all medicines in a locked cabinet out of the reach of young children. There are thousands of common household products which can kill if taken by mouth. Oven cleaners, antiseptics cosmetics, and lavatory cleaners are just a few examples. Unfortunately, not all poisons are clearly marked with a poison label or kept in a standard 'poison bottle' with ribbed sides like the one opposite. If any of these are taken the doctor should be called immediately.

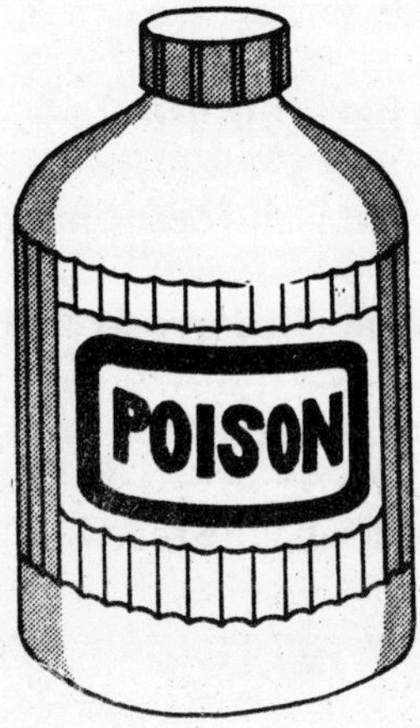

Dangerous plants

Another common source of poisons is the garden. The three poisonous plants illustrated below are just a few of the many attractive plants and berries to be found in your own back yard which can kill. If such berries or leaves are eaten, the victim should be encouraged to vomit. Recently weed killers such as paraquat and D.D.T. have been responsible for poisonings. These are dangerous substances. Never store them in lemonade bottles etc. where they might be found by children.

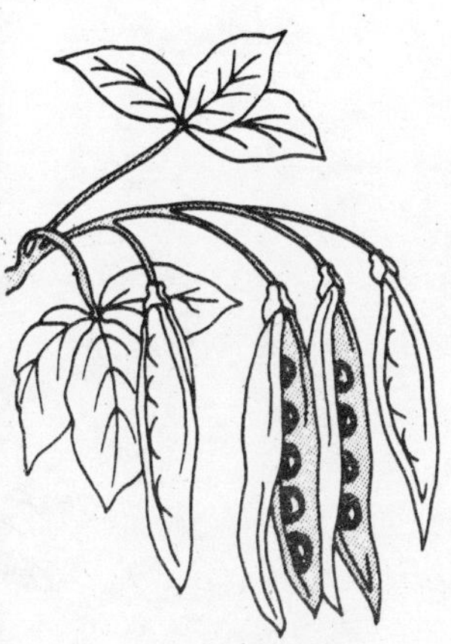

Laburnum
(*Laburnum Anagyroides*)

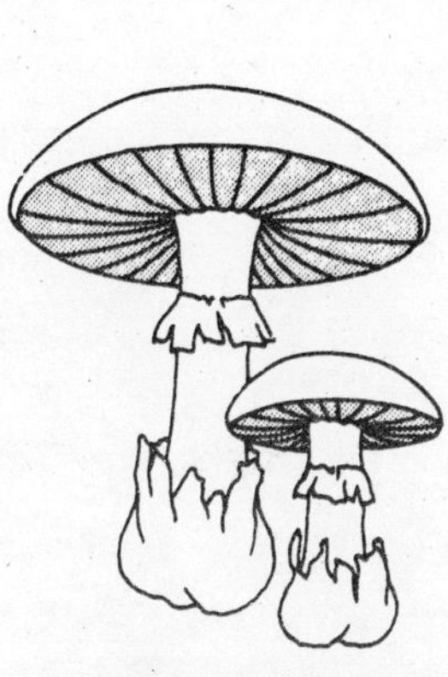

Death cap mushroom
(*Amanita Phalloides*)

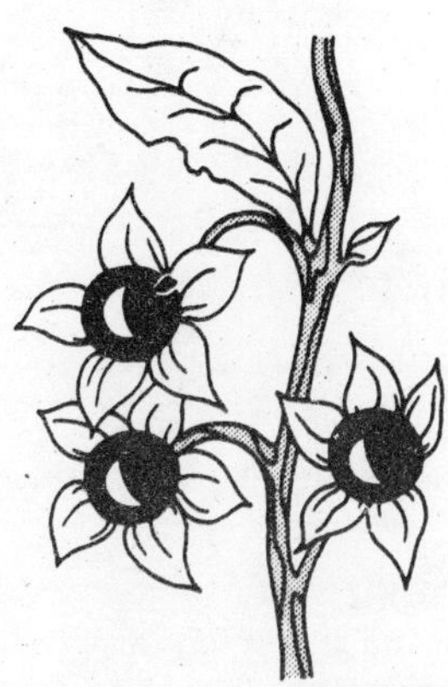

Deadly nightshade
(*Atropa Belladona*)

Quiz

1) What is a poison?

2) What is the oesophagus?

3) What is a corrosive poison? Describe the correct treatment for it.

4) What is stupor?

5) Describe the recovery position.

6) How can a poisoned person be made to vomit?

7) If the poisoned person is unconscious what should you do?

8) What should you do if the victim is not breathing?

9) What are the common sources of carbon monoxide?

10) How would you treat a wasp sting?

2 Coping with a burn

You are invited to a party to celebrate a friend's birthday. A lot of people turn up—one or two with guitars—and the room is soon crowded. During the evening a girl screams. She had been standing toc close to an unguarded fire and her nylon dress caught fire. A moment or two passes before you realise what is going on. By that time she is jumping up and down terrified.

What would you do to save her life?

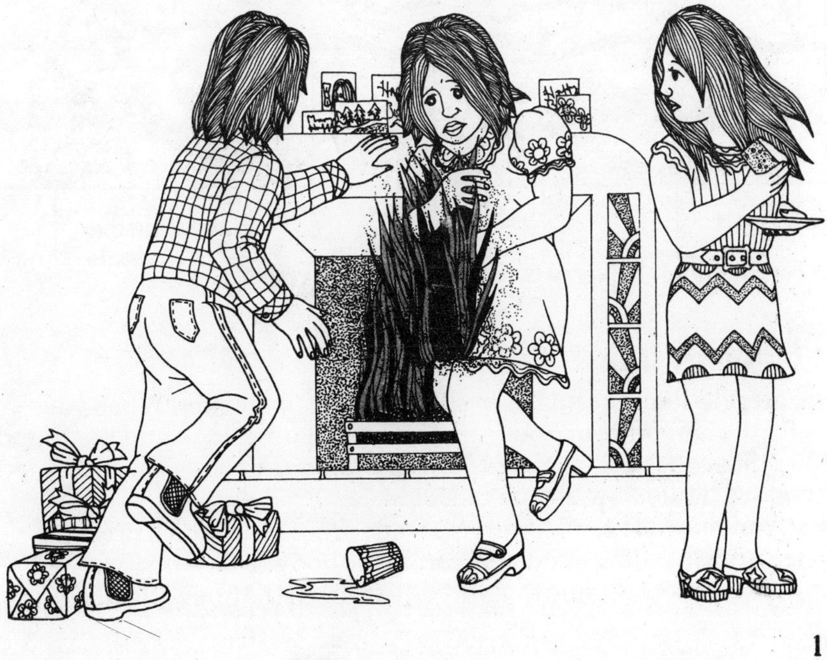

Theory

The skin: what is it made of?

The skin is the covering of the body. An essential organ which does many jobs, it is made up of three layers:

Epidermis: The top-most layer consisting of row upon row of slowly dying cells which give the skin a shiny waterproof surface.

Dermis: The sensitive part of the skin in which the touch and pain nerve endings are found. The dermis or live skin also contains many small sweat glands, fine hairs, muscles and blood vessels. Sweat, which is a salt and water solution, is lost from the skin.

Subcutaneous tissue: The bottom layer which contains fat, an insulating material, and larger blood vessels.

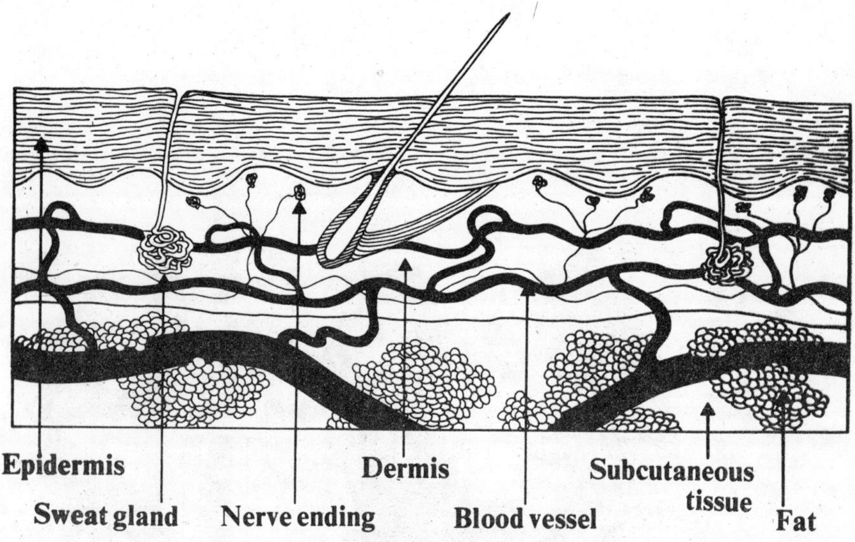

What does it do?

Heat regulation: The body is insulated by fat in the skin. When you shiver the hair on your body stands on end (goose flesh) and less blood flows through the skin. Heat is lost by evaporation of sweat and by increased blood flow through the skin.

Waterproofing: The epidermis is a waterproof layer which prevents water from invading or escaping from the body. This is of great importance considering that three quarters of the body is water.

Protection: The nerve endings in the dermis make us aware of dangerous situations by triggering off pain. For example, when you burn a finger it is the pain which warns you that the flame is touching the skin and causes you to pull your hand away. The skin also acts as a barrier to infection.

What is a burn?

Any area of the body from which skin has been removed by one of the following is said to be burned:

Dry heat: burn from cooking ring or fire
Electricity: from electric shock
Friction: a rope burn
Acids: hydrochloric acid (lavatory or oven cleaners)
Alkalis: soda lime
Radiation: following a large dose of deep x-ray treatment
Wet heat: boiling water or steam—usually called a scald

How deep does it go?

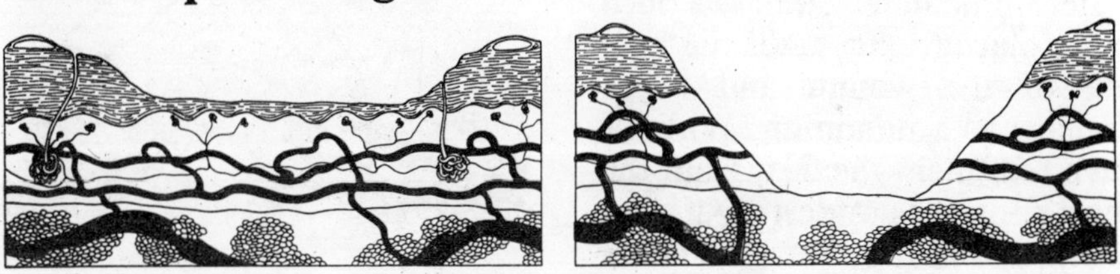

Superficial: In this type of burn only the epidermis, or top layer, is removed. It hurts but will eventually heal.

Deep: In a burn of this kind the epidermis and dermis are removed, as shown above. There is little or no pain but it will heal slowly and will leave a scar.

What does it look like?

Red raw skin
Blistering
Swelling in the immediate area
Oozing of fluid from the burn

How should it be treated?

The principle of treating a burn is to reduce heat caused by the burn; to prevent infection (by applying a sterile dressing) and to replace the fluid which has seeped from the body.

Step by Step

Remove cause of the burn

Smother the flames with a blanket or rug to exclude air and stop the burning.

Reduce heat

Soak the burnt part with cold water or a soothing fluid such as milk. This is most important, and at least 10 to 15 minutes should be spent on this step. The diagram below shows how damage from burns can be reduced by quick treatment. Soaking with cold water immediately after the burn takes place (right) takes the heat out of the wound and keeps damage to a minimum. Without such treatment the heat from the burn continues to destroy tissues and the resulting damage is much greater.

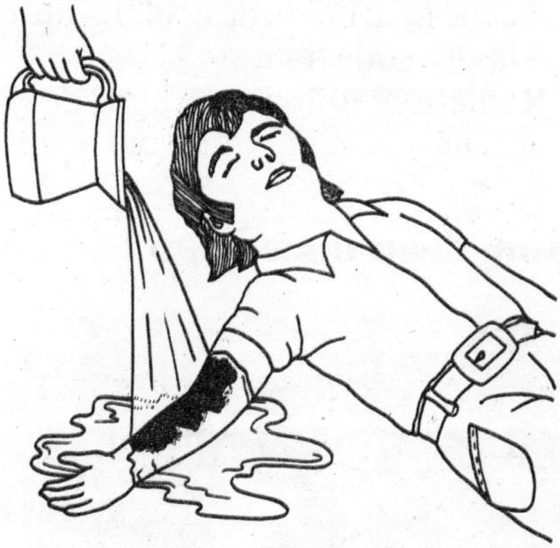

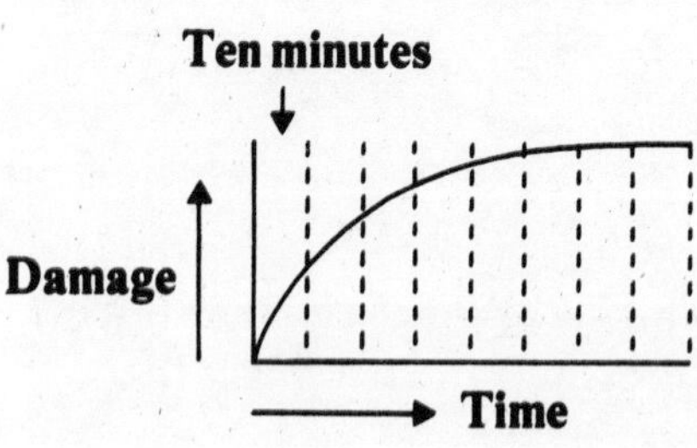

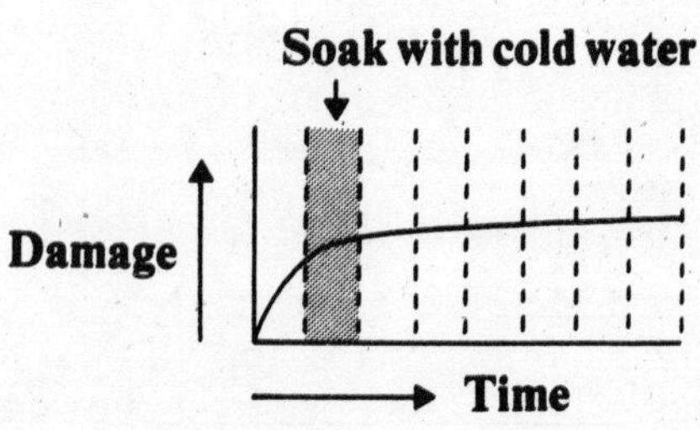

Remove rings

Rings or any constricting articles should be taken from the burned area. If this is not done, swelling may prevent the blood flowing properly.

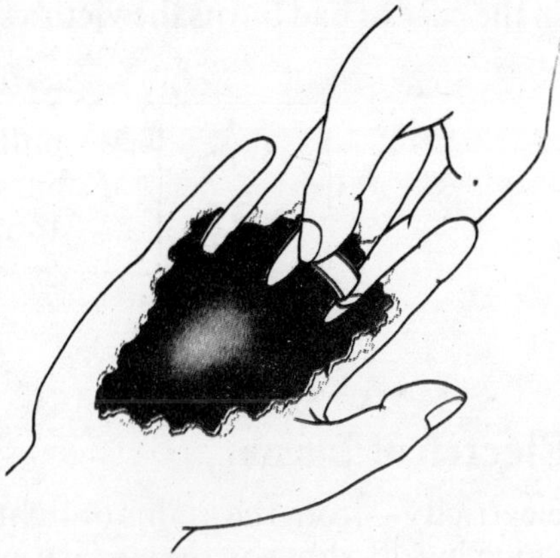

Apply a dressing

Apply the dressing as shown in Appendix 1. This will help stop infection entering the body through the damaged skin.

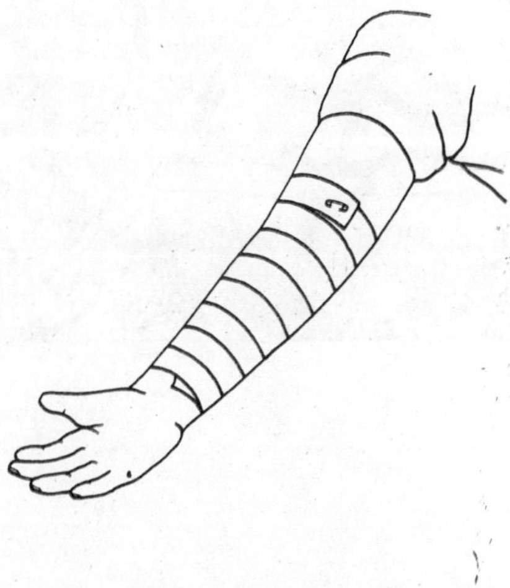

Restrict movement

If a part is badly burned, make sure it is not moved. Elevate to prevent further swelling.

Call an ambulance

In the case of bad burns the victim should be taken to hospital.

DO NOT	pull away burned skin burst blisters apply any ointment

Electrical burns

Electricity—from the mains or lightning—may produce deep burns which hardly show on the surface, as shown below.

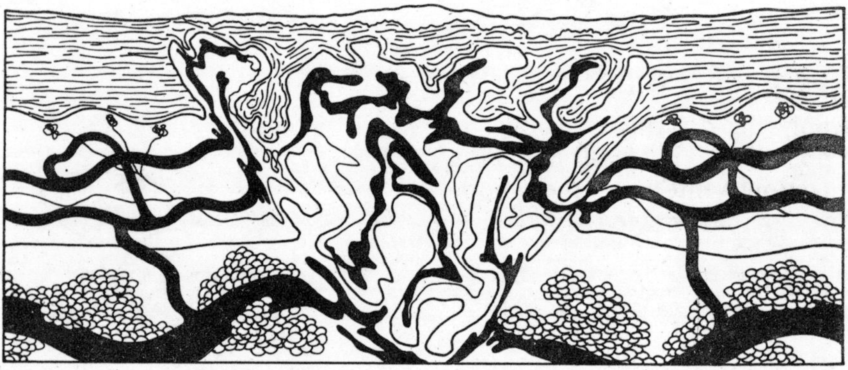

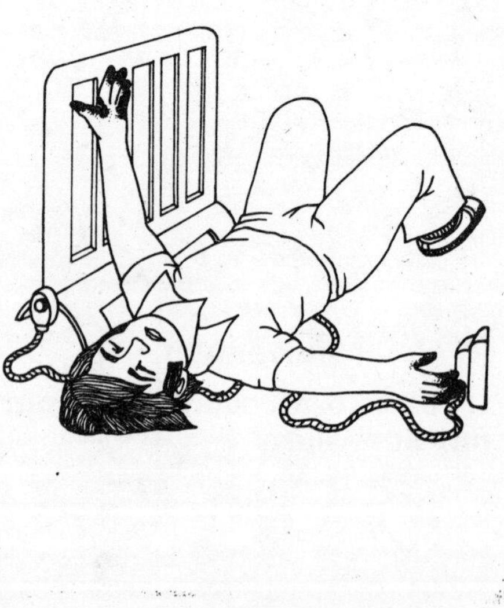

Electricity burns the point where it enters and where it leaves the body.
It may also cause the heart beat to fluctuate wildly and breathing to become irregular. Electric burns should be treated in the same way as ordinary burns.

Acid and alkaline burns

Any clothing which has been soaked by the chemical should be removed immediately. The burnt part should be thoroughly soaked with water and then wrapped in a dressing.

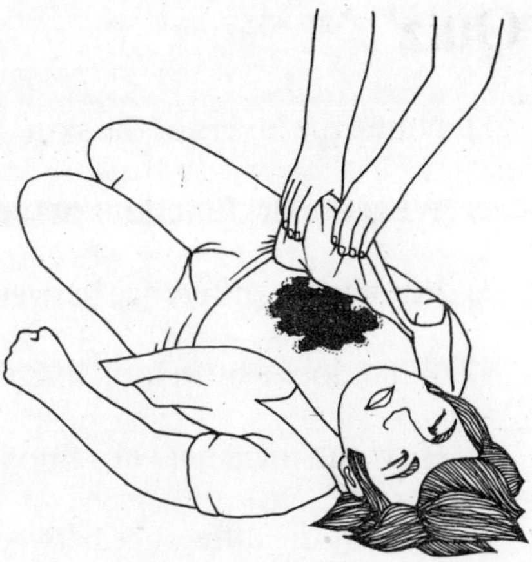

Burns to the mouth and throat

Dangerous swelling of the mouth and airways may be caused by burns in these areas, making it difficult to breathe. It is important to cool the burned area and reduce swelling with ice or cold water. Get medical help as soon as possible.

Burns to the eye

A burn to the eye may produce scarring and loss of sight. It is extremely important that any burns to the eye be dealt with immediately. Flush the burned area with water or milk. Dip the head into a bucket of water or wash basin. After at least ten minutes soaking put on a dressing and get medical help.

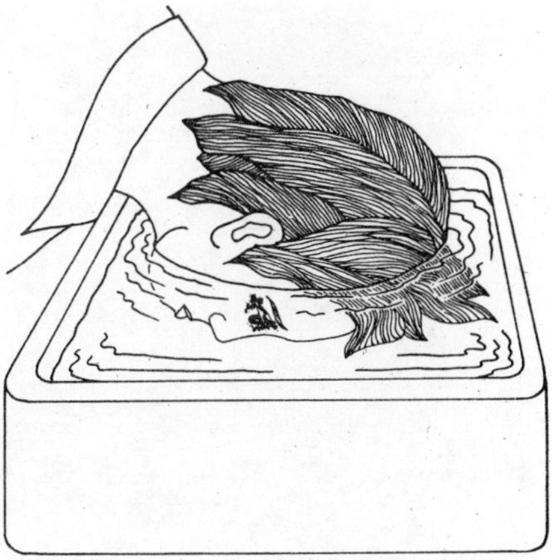

Sunburn

This is usually just on the surface (superficial). Apply a soothing liquid such as calamine lotion.

Quiz

1) Name the layers of the skin
2) What are the functions of the skin?
3) What is the difference between a burn and a scald?
4) What does a burn look like?
5) How can local heat be removed from a burned area?
6) What is the difference between deep and superficial burns?
7) Describe how you would treat a burn of the hand.
8) In what two places might you find electrical contact burns?
9) What is the special treatment of acid burns?
10) What is the special danger of burns to the mouth?

3 Out of joint?

Having checked your climbing equipment to make sure that you have everything you need, you set out with a group of potholers to explore underground caves. Several hours later you are working your way back to the surface when you hear a rumbling noise behind you. The roof of the cave is falling in and the last man in the team is likely to be trapped. A heavy rock falls on his leg before he has time to scramble out. You quickly lower yourself back down and try to pull him free. Eventually you move the boulder. He is still conscious but in great pain.

What would you do to save his life?

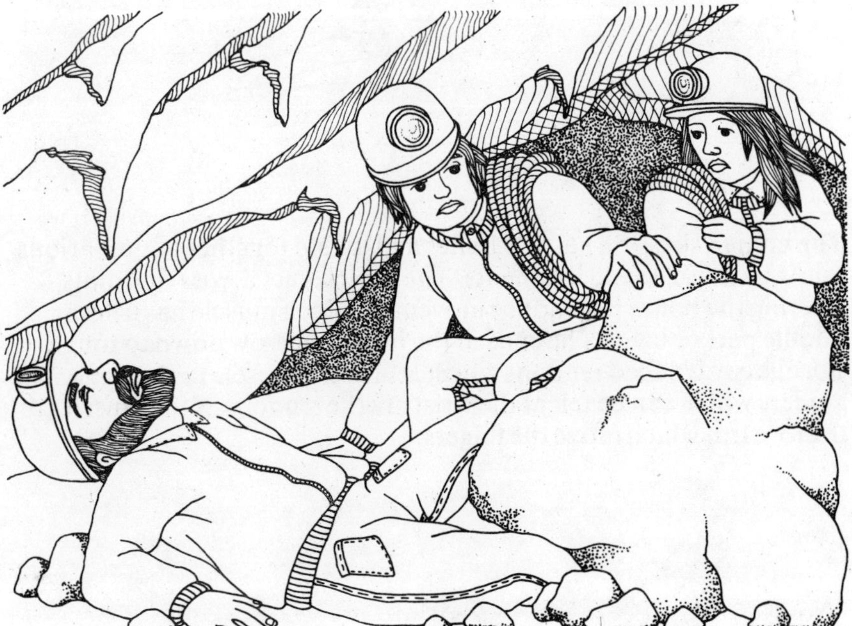

Theory

Injuries to muscles and joints commonly occur on the sportsfield and in other outdoor activities such as caving and mountaineering. Everyone who takes part in these sports should be able to cope with minor injuries that may happen. All damage to the soft tissue produces swelling, and all such injuries are treated in a similar way. The cold water sponge, often seen in the boxing ring and at football matches, is the secret of their treatment, as you will see in this chapter.

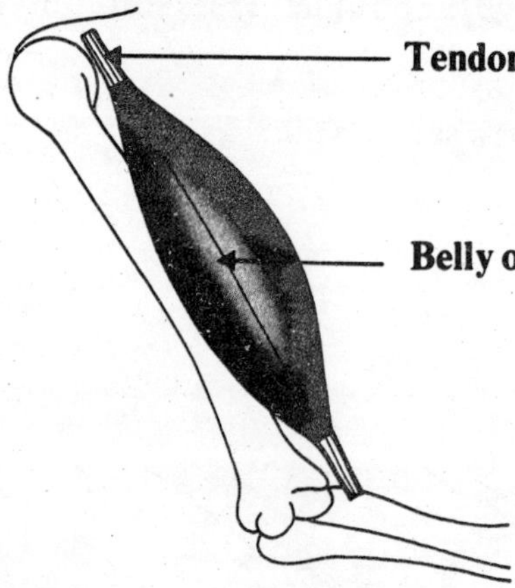

The human skeleton has 208 bones and is held together at the various joints by muscles and ligaments. The muscles act across the joints levering the bones to produce movement. Each muscle has a fleshy middle part or belly. The ends of the muscle narrow down to tough fibrous cords called tendons which attach the muscle to the bone. The guiders which can be felt at the wrist are the tendons of the muscles in the forearm which move the fingers.

Each muscle receives blood carrying essential oxygen and glucose, and this provides the energy necessary for shortening movement. Muscles are therefore red and will bleed if they are cut. They also have nerves which carry messages from the brain telling them when and how to move. Muscles may be damaged by being pulled (a muscle strain) or by being crushed.
Ligaments are tough fibrous bands which hold the ends of bones together at the joints. They cannot shorten and have no blood supply. They may be injured by being stretched or torn (a sprain).

Joints

Bones are joined together in various ways.

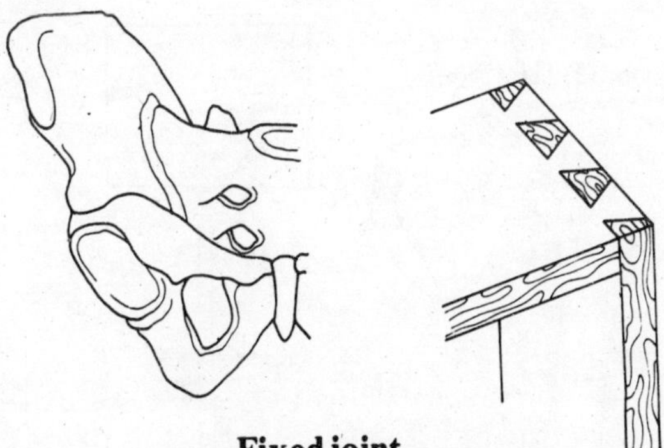

Fixed joint

Fixed joint: This is the simplest kind of joint where the bones are fixed together very tightly, for example, the bones of the skull or the pelvis. No movement is possible in this kind of joint. A fixed joint in the body is like a dovetail joint in wood.

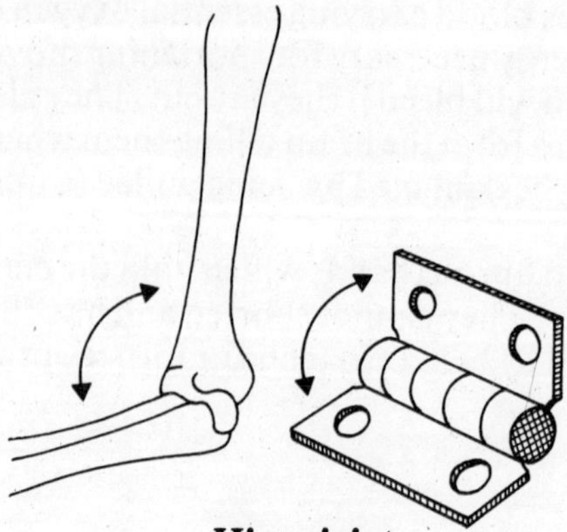

Hinge joint

Hinge joint: This is a joint where movement takes place in two opposite directions. Like the hinge of a door, these joints only open and close. Two examples are the knee joint and the elbow joint.

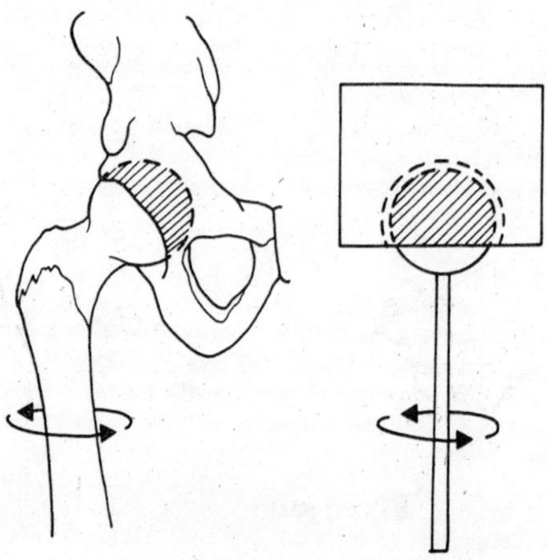

Ball and socket joint

Ball and socket joint: This is a joint which allows movement in many directions. It is the biological example of a universal joint, used in the gear lever of a car. The hip and shoulder joints are such joints.

When the two bone ends which form a joint lose contact with each other the bones are said to be out of joint or the joint dislocated. Several joints in the body contain small pieces of cartilage (gristle) which lessen the wear and tear on the bone ends. This cartilage may tear and come out of place or dislocate.

Each of these injuries produce swelling and pain. The basic treatment is to reduce the swelling and lessen the pain. This is done by cooling, bandaging and lifting up the injured part, or:

Ice or cold water held on the injury

Compression of the swelling with a firmly applied bandage

Elevation of the injured limb

Crush injury

If a muscle is trapped under a heavy weight for a long time it will be badly injured and parts of the muscle will die. The dead tissue produces poisonous chemicals which are carried by the blood to the kidneys. Eventually, the kidneys may stop working. The injured muscle swells and becomes painful and red.
No time should be lost in treating a crush injury. The trapped muscles must be freed quickly and the injured limb rested. Movement encourages the release of the dangerous chemicals. The victim must be taken to hospital quickly because an operation may be needed. Do not give the victim anything to drink.

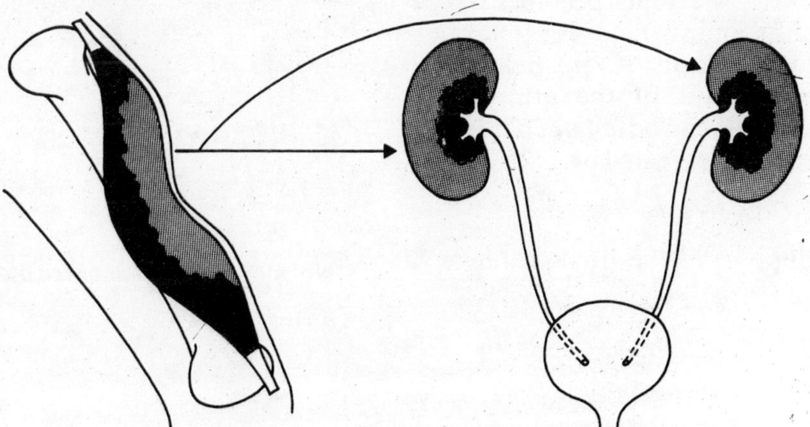

Crush injury to muscle involves the kidneys

Step by Step

Dislocated cartilage

The type of cartilage which is most often found torn is the inside cartilage of the knee. It may happen, for example, when a footballer turns suddenly. The joint becomes tender and swollen, is painful to move and may 'lock' which means that although it bends easily it will not straighten without producing severe pain. A torn cartilage should be treated by:

Reducing swelling

Supporting the injured leg with soft padding between and under the knee

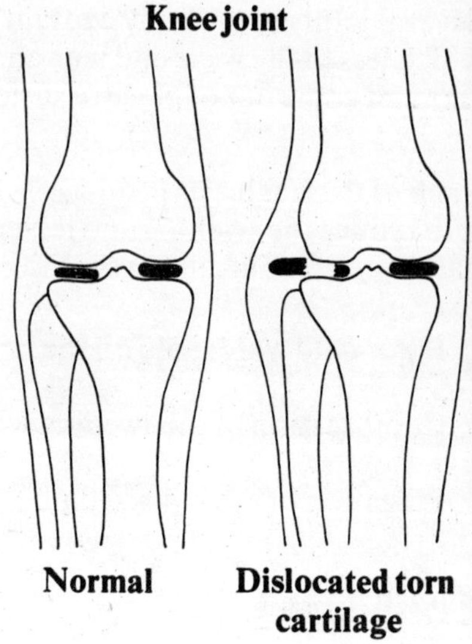

Dislocated joint

The shoulder is a freely movable joint which may come out of its socket. The joint becomes very painful and swollen. It cannot be moved without severe pain and the top end of the arm bone (humerus) can be felt out of place. It should be treated by:

Reducing local swelling

Supporting the arm in a sling

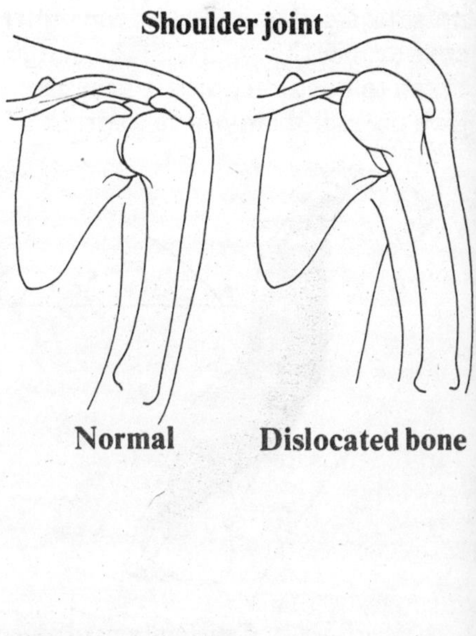

A sprain

Sudden movement, such as twisting the foot on a kerbstone, may stretch or tear the ankle ligaments. This produces a painful swollen joint which is unstable because of the stretched ligament. It is often very difficult to tell the difference between a severe sprain and a fracture of the bone. But this is not important because the first aid treatment is the same for both cases:

Reduction of local swelling

Firm support of the injured joint by immobilising the joint with padding and broad bandages

Ankle joint

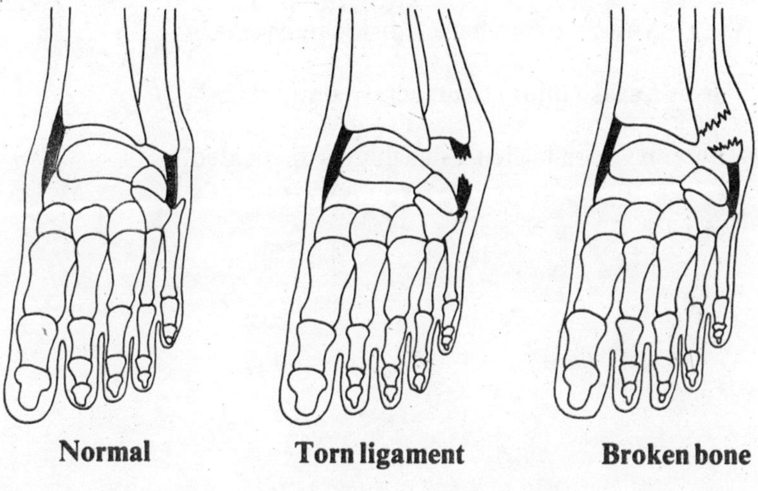

A strain

Sudden severe pulling of a muscle produces local bruising and swelling in the muscle—a muscular strain. The muscle is painful, tender and swollen. Cold water or ice should be applied, followed by a firm bandage and a period of rest until the swelling subsides.

Quiz

1) What kind of joints are there in the body?

2) What is the difference between a ligament and a tendon?

3) Does a joint cartilage have any useful purpose?

4) Write out the basic treatment of a soft tissue injury.

5) What is a strain and how is it different from a sprain?

6) How can you tell if a knee cartilage is torn?

7) If you are unable to decide if there is a fracture as well as a soft tissue injury, what would you do?

8) Should you try to put back a dislocated joint?

9) Why is a crush injury to muscle so dangerous?

10) How can you tell when a shoulder is dislocated?

4 If a bone breaks

A few days after new neighbours move in at the bottom of your street you notice the father of the family out painting window frames. At first he takes great care, moving the ladder each time a frame is out of reach. But, as daylight fades he is rushing to finish the job and stretches to paint a small window at the top of the house. Suddenly, he loses his balance and topples off the ladder. He falls on to the concrete below and does not move.

What would you do to save his life?

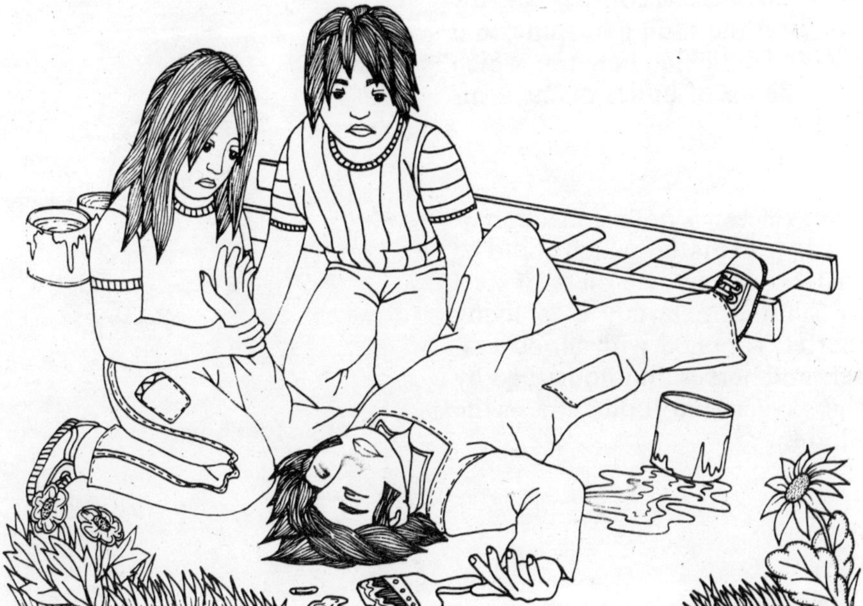

Bones come in different shapes and sizes but each has features by which it can be identified. There are three basic shapes:

Long bones: such as the bones of the arm or leg.

Short bones: the bones of the wrist or backbone (vertebral column).

Flat bones: such as the bones of the skull or pelvis.

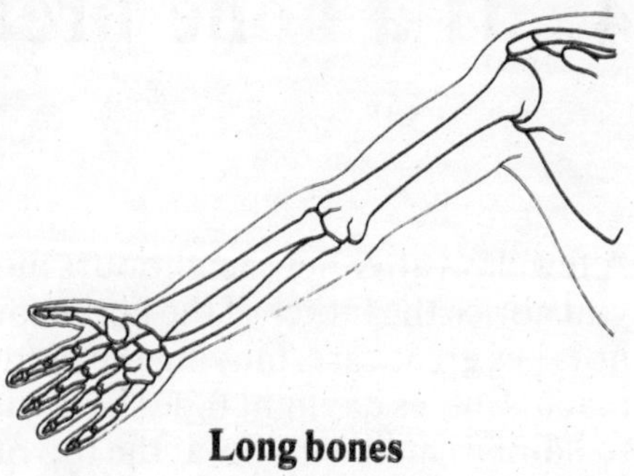

Long bones

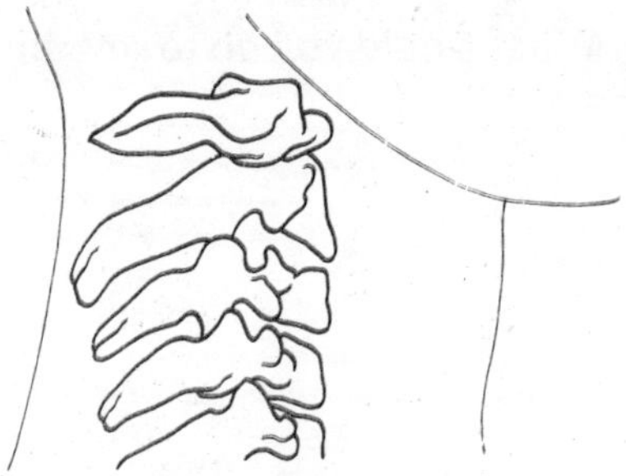

Short bones

There are 208 bones in the human skeleton and these are all joined together by ligaments and muscles. The skeleton has two main parts; the central or axial skeleton which consists of the bones of the skull and spine, and the appendicular skeleton which is made up of bones of the arms and legs.

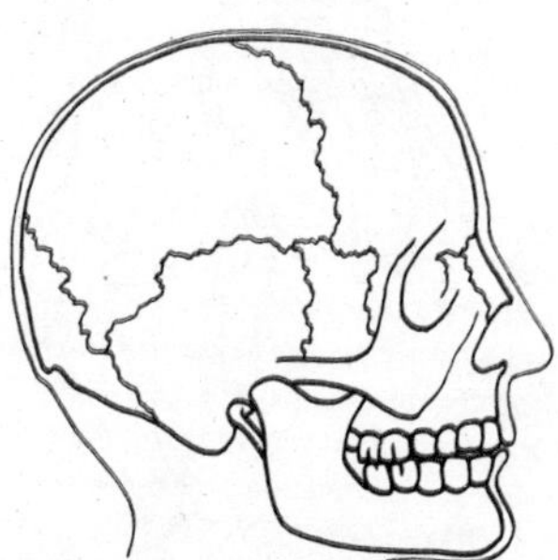

Flat bones

The skeleton is not a collection of hard, dead matter which could be easily replaced by a piece of steel or similar material; it is living matter, supplied with blood vessels and nerves and nourished by the oxygen and foodstuffs in the blood.

The skeleton has three main functions:

Form and movement: it provides a frame for the body. It also supports the soft tissue and is clothed by muscles. These stretch across joints and hold two or more bones together. When a muscle stretches it pulls bones nearer to each other and, in this way, produces movement.

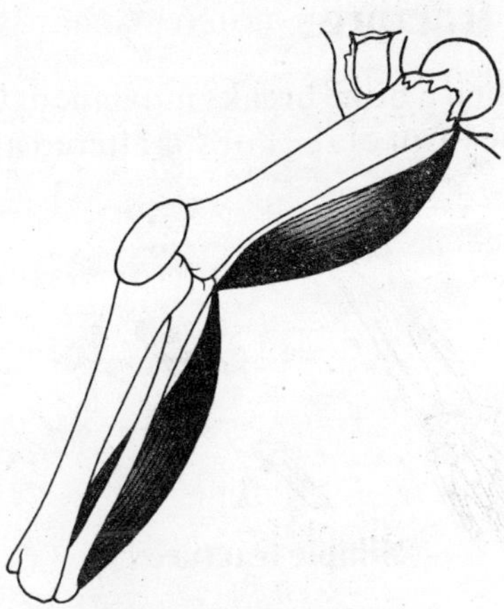

Bones and movement

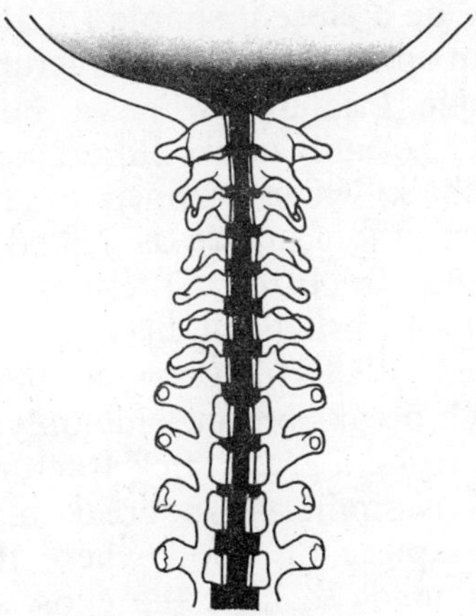

Bones and safety

Protection: bones serve to give protection to vital bodily organs. For example, the soft tissue of the brain is encased within the hard skull bones; the delicate spinal cord is sheathed by a tunnel of connected backbones; the heart and lungs are protected by the rib cage.

Blood formation: bones are important living material. The soft jelly-like marrow in the centre of the hard, outer layer of bone is particularly vital because it manufactures blood cells.

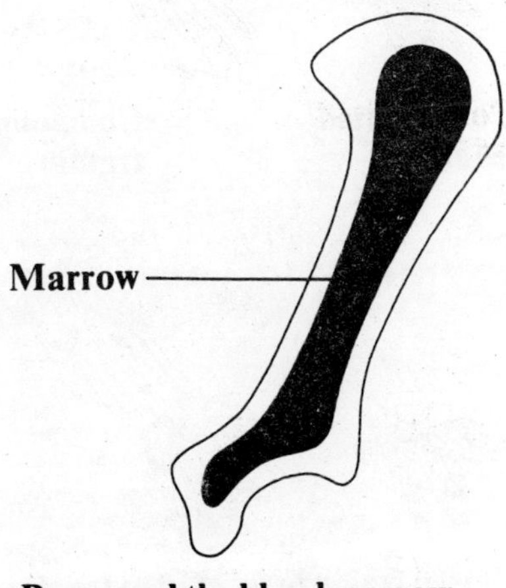

Bones and the blood marrow

A fracture

When a bone breaks movement becomes difficult and painful. The form of the body is altered and takes on an abnormal shape at the point of the break. A bone which is broken is said to be fractured or cracked. There are different types of fractures and these are listed below. The names are unimportant in themselves but they do serve as a guide to the damage which may be caused by a particular fracture. Any fracture may be described by several of these terms. For example; a break may be a closed, simple fracture or an open, complicated fracture.

Simple fracture: when a bone breaks cleanly in two (like a piece of chalk when dropped on the floor), the fracture is called a simple fracture. Fractures in adults are usually of this kind.

Green stick fracture: a bone which breaks on one side only is said to be a green stick fracture. This is similar to a break in a green piece of wood where the bark tends to hold the ends together.

Complicated and compound fractures: a fracture is termed complicated when the broken ends of the bone tear into other parts of the body such as blood vessels or nerves. Fractures are compound when there is more than one break in the same bone.

Open and closed fractures: when the broken ends of bone puncture the skin and are exposed the fracture is known as "open". If the skin is undamaged then the fracture is said to be "closed".

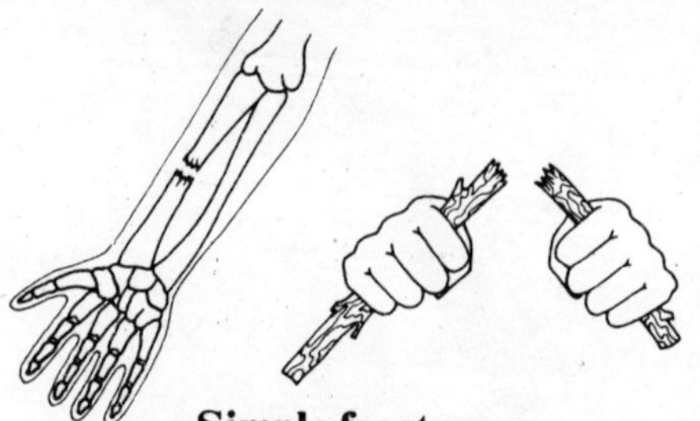

Simple fracture

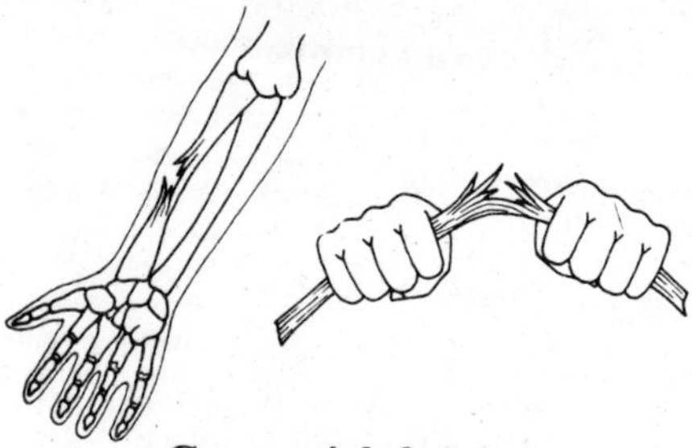

Green stick fracture

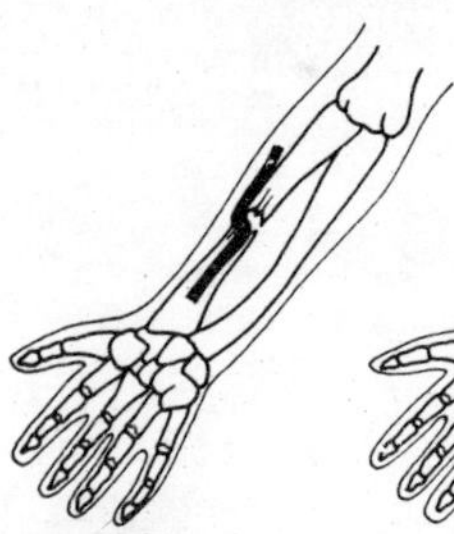

Complicated fracture

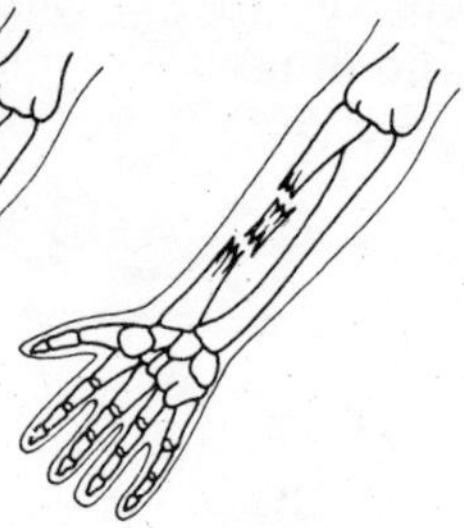

Compound fracture

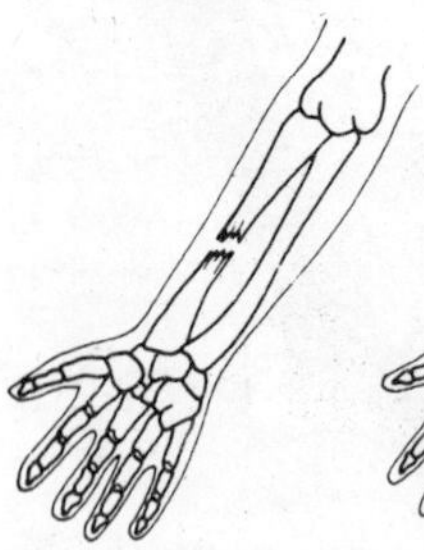

Closed fracture

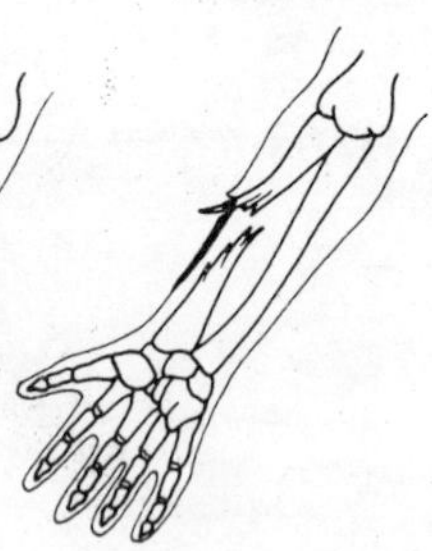

Open fracture

What does a fracture look like?

The identifying signs of a fracture may be remembered by the word PULSE:

Pain

Unusual shape

Loss of use

Swelling and tenderness

Extra movement

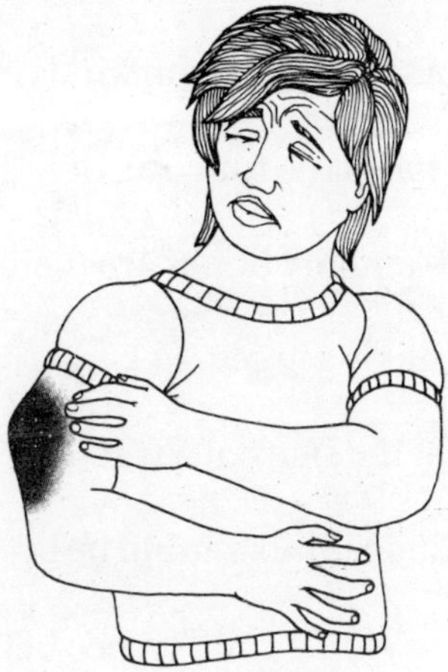

Fractured arm

Treatment

A fracture heals when the broken ends manufacture new bone to cement the break. In order for this process to be effective the bone ends must be held together for a period of time, from a few weeks to months, depending on the site and type of break, and the age and condition of the victim. This is best done by putting a plaster cast around the limb or screwing the bones together with a metal plate. The First-Aider should immobilize the limb to prevent the broken ends from causing pain or further damage. To do this, the joints above and below the break must be prevented from moving. (For example, if the bones of the lower leg are broken the knee and ankle must be immobilized.) In this way, the muscles attached to the broken bone will not be able to shorten and pull the ends apart.

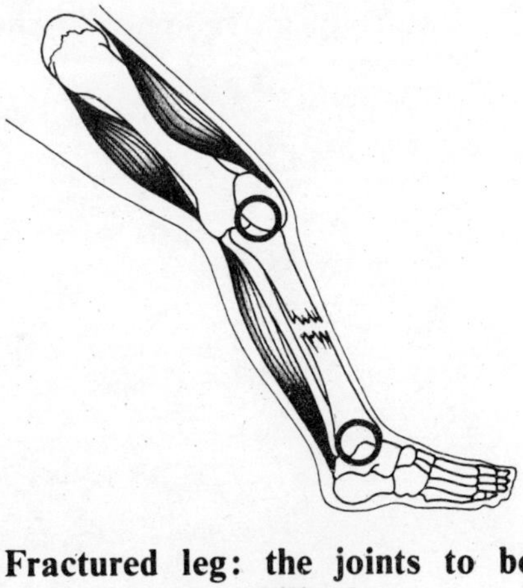

Fractured leg: the joints to be immobilised.

The treatments of the various fractures are explained in Appendix 2.

Quiz

1) Name the different kinds of bones.

2) What is the function of bone marrow?

3) How many bones are there in the body?

4) What is a greenstick fracture?

5) List the signs of a fracture.

6) Which joints should be immobilised if the arm is broken?

7) Describe the difference between a complicated and compound fracture.

8) What are the functions of the skeleton?

9) Give the difference between a simple and closed fracture.

10) Would you move someone who had fallen and was unconscious?

5 It's a knockout

It is a warm sunny day in the middle of summer term. Your school cricket team is playing the boys' grammar school in a one day championship match. The game is nearly over and your team only needs five runs to win. Time is running short when your batsman tries to hit a bouncer. He misses and the cricket ball smashes him on the forehead. He falls unconscious to the ground.

What would you do to save his life?

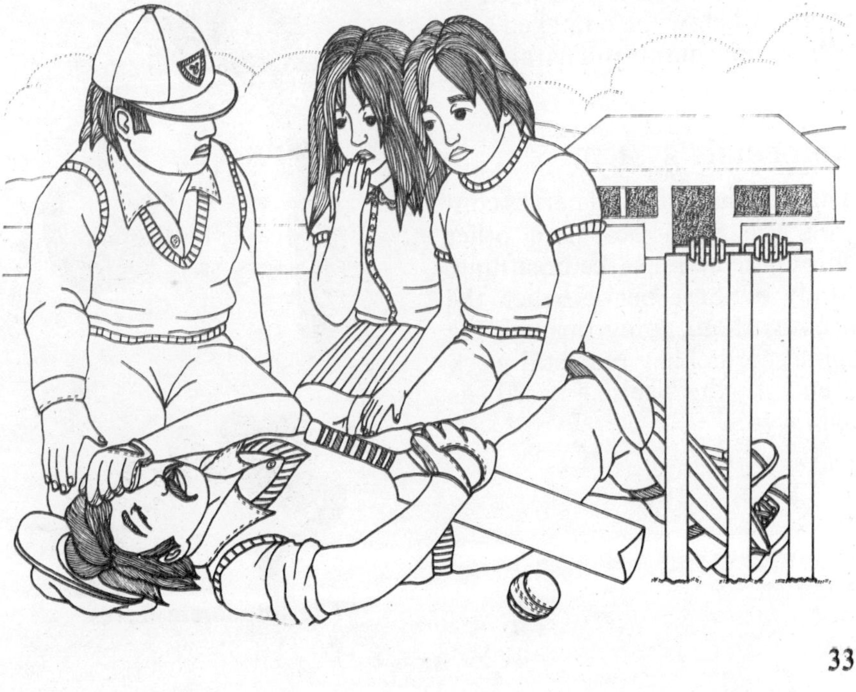

Theory

There are two basic systems of nerves in the body: cerebro spinal and autonomic, and an injury to either can be serious.

Cerebro-spinal system

The brain is made up of millions of nerves which control our physical and mental activities. Instructions are sent out to the body from it by a type of nerve (motor nerve) which switches on our muscles to produce movement. In the same way messages about the things around us—the air we breathe, the objects we touch, etc.—are sent to the brain through the sensory nerves. All these nerves travel to or from the brain through the spinal cord. If the spinal cord is injured parts of the body below the damaged area will become numb and paralysed.

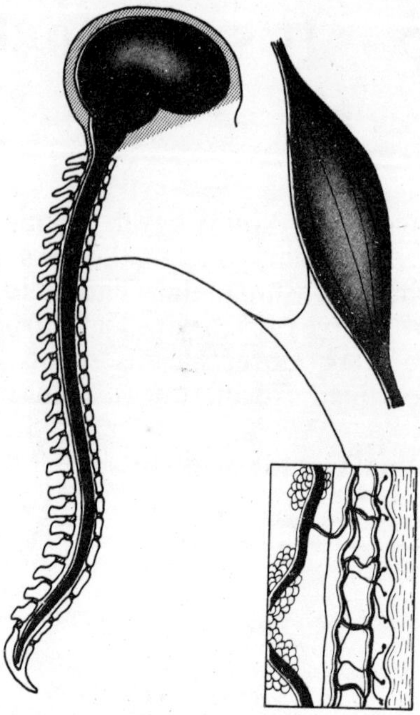

The cerebro spinal nerves

Autonomic system

This second system of nerves controls the heart beat and other automatic actions like breathing. Many of these nerves reach the brain without going through the spinal cord. They may still work even if the spinal cord is damaged.

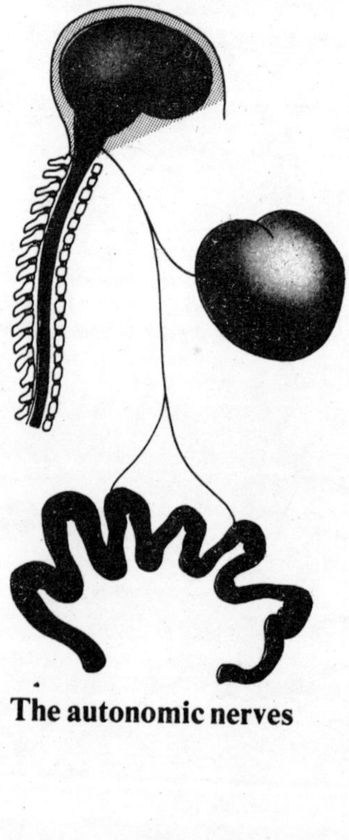

The autonomic nerves

Blood supply

The brain and spinal cord are supplied by blood vessels which deliver blood to the nervous tissue. The brain needs oxygen and sugar to function properly. If the blood supply is cut off and oxygen and sugar do not reach the brain it will stop working.

Protection

Very soft and easily damaged, the brain is encased by the skull bones which protect it from injury. A layer of fluid reduces the vibration of the brain within the skull and this layer acts as a biological shock absorber. The spinal cord is also encased in this fluid. It runs down a canal in the back bones (vertebral column) and is protected by them.

Stages of unconsciousness

Any person who has been knocked out is said to be unconscious. Progress of unconscious victims is measured in the following four stages:

I Fully conscious: awake and can talk sensibly.
II Drowsy: awake at times but seems to dose off. Speech is slurred.
III Stupor: will wake up only if severe pain is inflicted.
IV Coma: cannot be woken up.

It is important to know what stage of unconsciousness the victim is in throughout the period of care so that his progress can be assessed correctly. If he becomes drowsy and sinks into stupor or even coma, his condition is worsening and immediate medical help should be sought. When there is improvement there is less urgency.

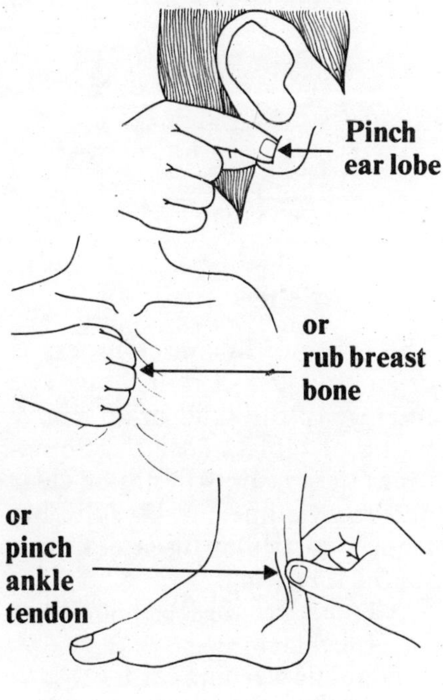

How conscious is the victim?

Step by Step

Any unconscious victim is in danger of suffocation (obstructed breathing) by his own tongue blocking the airway at the back of the mouth. He may vomit and because he has no control over swallowing while unconscious it may run down the airway into the windpipes and choke him. To avoid this, place the victim in the recovery position with the head pulled back and the jaw pushed forward as illustrated below. It is essential to feel the pulse and check the breathing. If either of these is faltering, then external cardiac compression or mouth to mouth resuscitation should be started. Send for medical help.

The recovery position

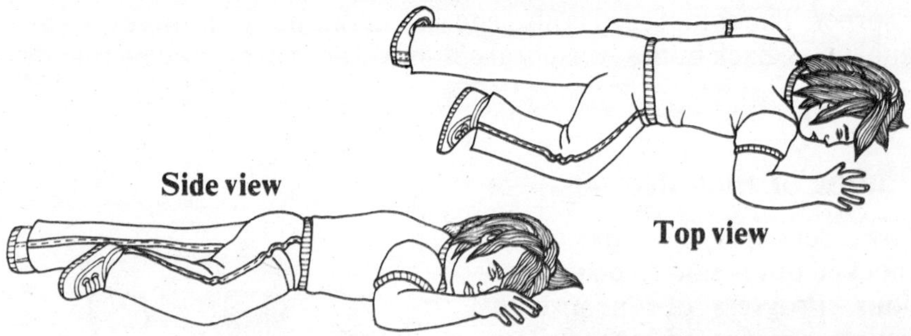

Finding the cause

The cause of unconsciousness is often obvious—a scalp wound or fracture of the skull or an empty bottle of tablets near by. Sometimes the reason will not be clear and the victim may be suffering from a particular disease. Check for the following:

- Medic-alert bracelet or disc (necklace)
- Diabetic warning cards
- Anticoagulant warning cards
- Epileptic warning cards
- Steroid warning cards

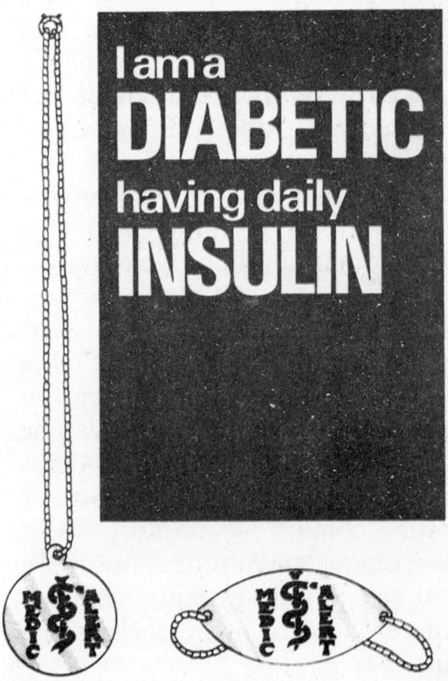
I am a
DIABETIC
having daily
INSULIN
MEDIC ALERT
MEDIC ALERT

These often give instructions for emergency treatment which should be followed. If a warning card or medic-alert disc is found it should be handed to the doctor or ambulance crew.

Head injury

A bang in the head may cause various injuries:

Brain concussion: This occurs when the brain vibrates or shakes within the skull. It temporarily interferes with brain activity and often causes loss of memory and coma. Breathing is shallow and shock may develop. If the victim falls into coma he should be placed in the recovery position and an ambulance called. If the victim regains consciousness, he should be told to seek medical help in case brain compression develops.

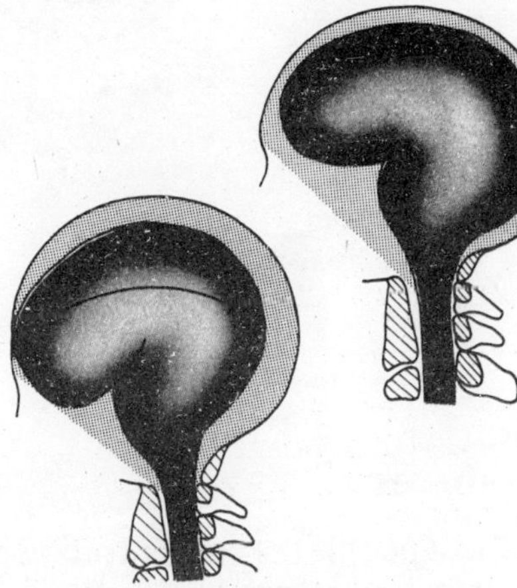

Brain concussion (shaking)

Brain compression: This can be caused by a depressed (sunk in) fracture of the skull pressing on the brain (see diagram) or by a blood clot between the skull and the brain (see diagram). A blood clot can take some time to develop and the first signs of brain compression may not appear immediately. A person suffering from brain compression usually breathes with difficulty and is flushed in the face. The part of the brain which is compressed does not function properly and part of the body becomes numb and/or paralysed. The victim will

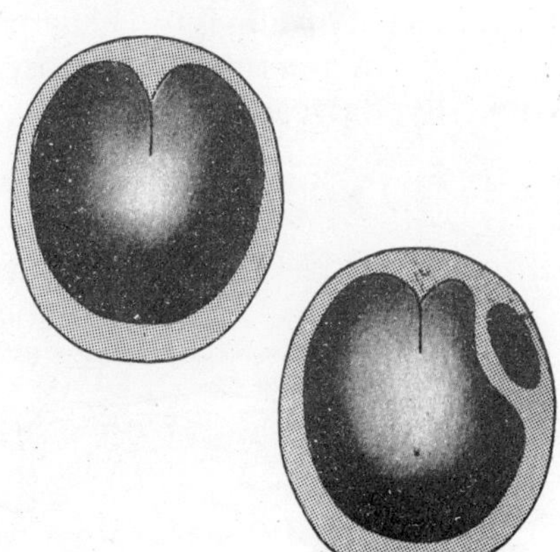

Brain compression (bleeding)

become unconscious and should be placed in the recovery position. Send for medical help immediately.

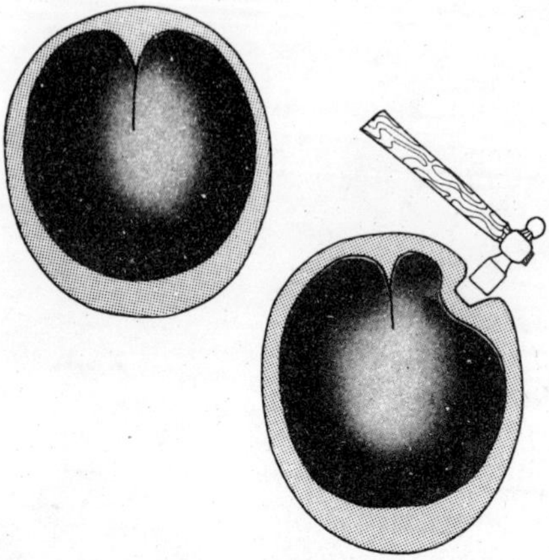

Brain compression (fracture)

Diabetes

In most people the concentration of sugar in the blood is regulated by a chemical substance called insulin. Diabetics have insufficient insulin to prevent a build up of sugar, and if it becomes too high they will lose consciousness. This condition is called diabetic coma (hyperglycaemia). It is treated by a doctor with insulin injections.
If the dose of insulin is too high or if no sugar is eaten, the blood sugar becomes low and the diabetic loses consciousness. This is called insulin coma (hypoglycaemia).

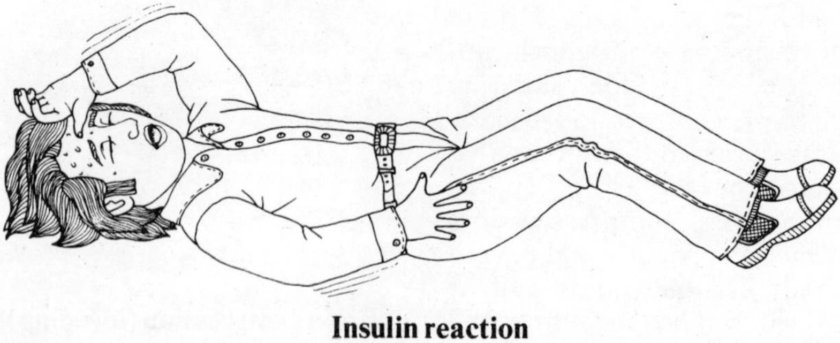

Insulin reaction

Diabetic coma: This condition occurs only among badly controlled diabetics and first-aiders are not likely to meet it often. It comes on slowly over several days and the diabetic becomes very ill. He often has a smell of nail varnish or pear drops or over-ripe apples on his breath (acetone). There is little that you can do for the victim. Put him in the recovery position and call medical help.

Insulin coma: This type of coma comes on quickly—usually just before a meal—and it is the diabetic problem which first-aiders are more likely to have to deal with. The victim is often angry and difficult to talk to. He may appear to be drunk but there will be no smell of alcohol. Treat this insulin reaction with two tablespoons of sugar in water. You will probably find sugar in his pocket or bag. If he is not given sugar immediately he will quickly become unconscious (insulin coma). In this case place the victim in the recovery position and call a doctor or ambulance. While waiting for the ambulance or doctor put a sugar lump or teaspoonful of sugar in the mouth. A little of this sugar will get into the blood and help the victim. Of course no attempt should be made to make an unconscious victim swallow sugar.

When in doubt: If you are not certain which type of illness the diabetic is suffering from, treat as insulin reaction.
Give sugar if the victim is *not* unconscious.

Epilepsy

The brain cells work by a form of biological electricity. Occasionally this electrical system goes wrong and everything discharges at once. This produces an epileptic attack or 'fit'. There are two main types of epileptic fit—major and minor (grand mal and petit mal).

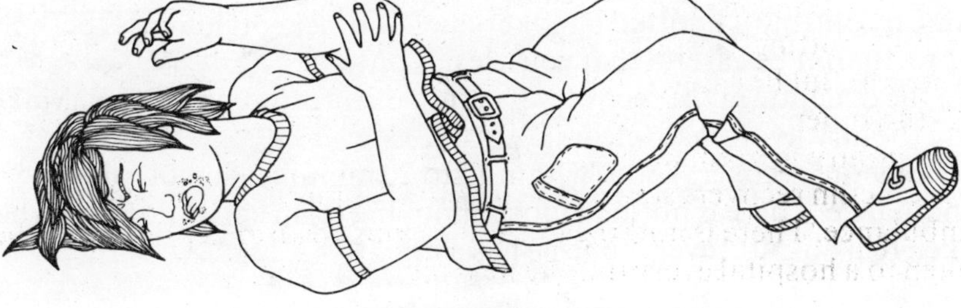

Epileptic fit

Minor epilepsy (Petit Mal): This usually occurs in children and is nothing more than a short loss of consciousness. It is often so brief that the child looks simply dazed or distant and may not even fall over. There can be many such fits during the day and children get so used to this they carry on as though nothing has happened.

Major epilepsy (Grand Mal): This is a much more serious condition and takes place in the following order:

Aura—a short warning that a fit is about to happen. It lasts a few seconds or may not occur at all. There is often no time to do anything about it.

Rigid stage—the victim tightens all his muscles and falls to the ground. He may cry out as all the air is forced from his lungs and he may pass water or open his bowels. He does not breathe and may go blue in the face. This stage lasts only about half a minute so it is not necessary to start mouth to mouth resuscitation. In any case the muscles are so tight that it is impossible to blow air into the lungs.

Shaking stage—this is known as the convulsion. The victim shakes violently. Even the jaw vibrates and the victim may hurt his tongue. After several minutes this stops.

Coma stage—after the convulsion, the epileptic often stays quietly unconscious for about half an hour. During this time he may vomit or obstruct his breathing.

What to do: Try to prevent injury when the victim falls.
Stop the victim biting his tongue during the shaking stage. This is best done by putting a knotted handkerchief or other soft material between the teeth. But be careful that you are not bitten.
Put the epileptic in the recovery position during the coma stage. Make sure the airways remain clear.
If the victim recovers soon (within 15 to 20 minutes) do not call an ambulance. There is nothing more annoying to an epileptic than to be taken to a hospital every time he has a fit.

Hysterical reactions

These are caused by an emotional condition which the victim does not understand. The reaction may vary from a temper tantrum to a state which looks like epilepsy. Such fits are dramatic and almost always occur in public. Treat the victim with kindness.

Gentle and firm reassurance may be sufficient but if the victim seems unconscious place in the recovery position.

Stroke (apoplexy)

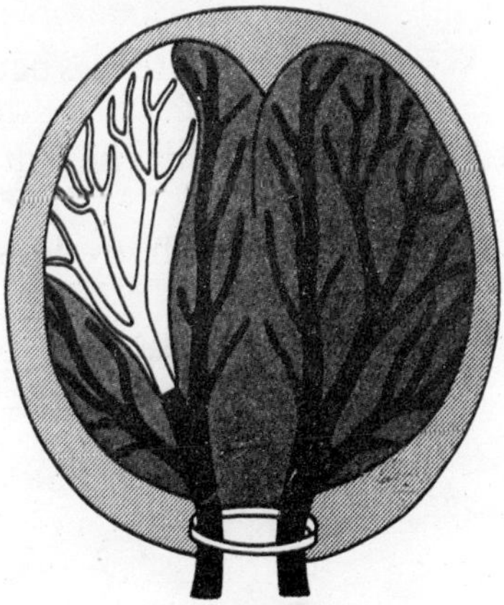

The brain is supplied with blood by a system of blood vessels which after a certain point do not connect with each other. If one of these blood vessels bursts or is blocked, then the part of the brain which it supplies will not receive sufficient blood and will stop working. This usually happens in older people.

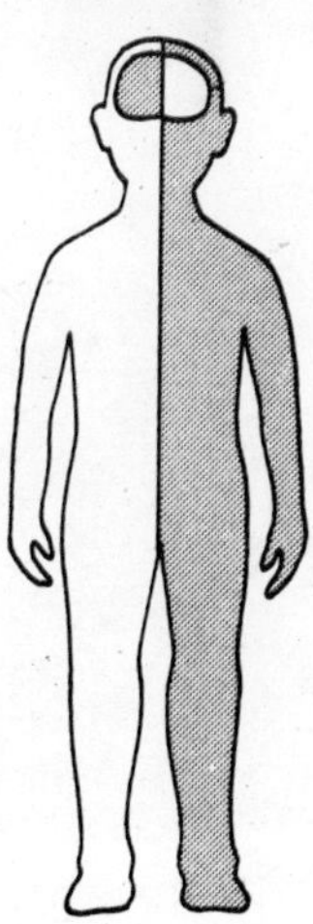

The right side of the brain controls the left side of the body, and vice versa. If the left side of the brain is short of blood then the right side or part of the right side will not work correctly. It may become numb or paralysed or both. If the area of the brain is large or if certain regions of it are affected, then the victim will become unconscious. There is very little that the First-Aider can do in this situation. Place the victim in the recovery position and call medical help as soon as possible.

Quiz

1) What is the cerebro-spinal system of nerves?

2) Describe stupor and how would you test the level of unconsciousness?

3) Where would you find a medic-alert disc?

4) What is the difference between brain compression and brain concussion?

5) What is an insulin coma?

6) What is the treatment of an insulin reaction?

7) What are the differences between epileptic and hysterical fits?

8) Should all epileptics be sent to hospital after having a fit?

9) Which half of the body does the left side of the brain control?

10) What is a stroke?

6 How to survive

You are walking on Dartmoor when you discover an unconscious man. He had set out the previous day on a 30-kilometre hike without any preparation and not giving much thought to the weather. On the way strong winds began blowing and it started raining. Without waterproof clothing the hiker was soon soaked to the skin. At first he was irritated and annoyed at being caught in the open. Then his condition gradually got worse and the pleasant open-air excursion turned into a nightmare of exposure. He slowed down, became clumsy, his vision blurred and he began stumbling about drunkenly. He shivered violently as his body temperature dropped. Finally, with his built-in heat control no longer working, he collapsed.

What would you do to save his life?

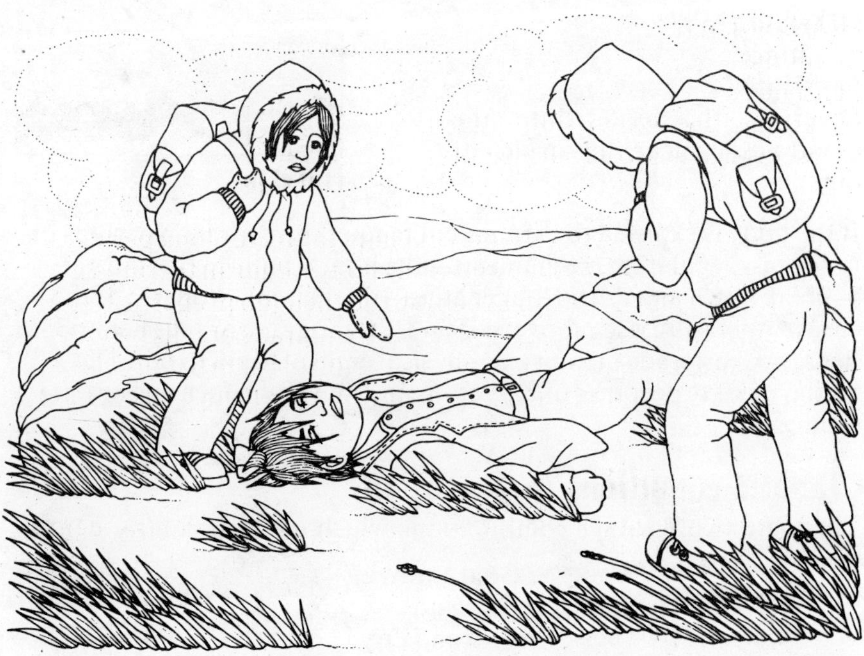

Theory

Every year there are many cases like that of the hiker. People—young and old—climb hills or mountains or set out on long walks without proper clothing or equipment. The weather changes suddenly and soon they are suffering from cold exhaustion, frostbite or even severe hypothermia. Others fail to take precautions against the sun and are struck down by heat exhaustion or heat stroke. This chapter explains these various conditions and how to survive them.

Temperature control

Although the surface or skin temperature of the body often changes, the inner core—the brain and trunk—remains constant at 37 degrees Centigrade.

This happens in several ways:

Heat is maintained by:
Chemical reactions in the body and exercise.
Shivering.
Directing the blood away from the blood vessels in the skin.

Heat is lost by:
Sweating.
Panting.
Diverting the blood into the blood vessels near the surface of the skin.

Temperature changes and the skin

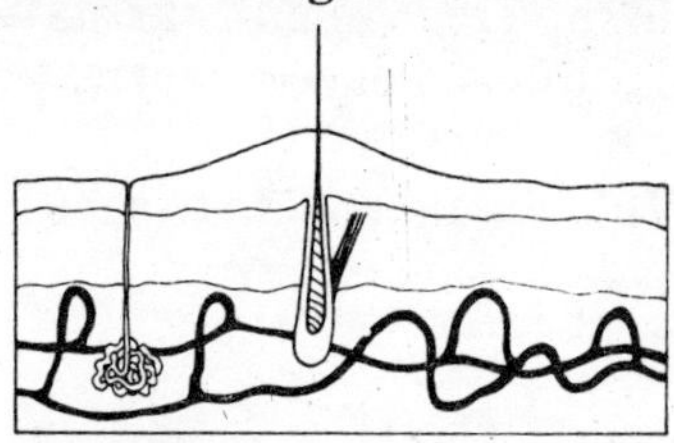

Cold skin

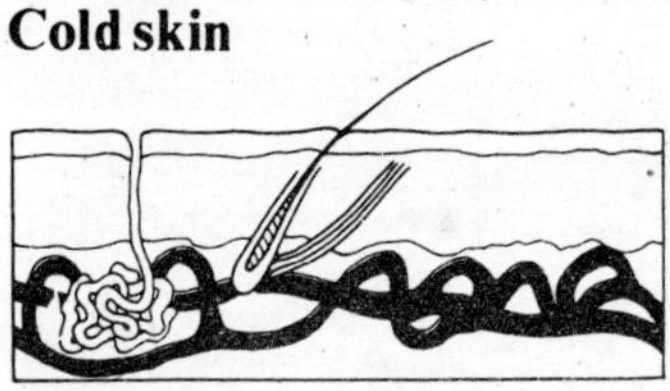

Hot skin

If the body is exposed to extremes of temperature for long periods of time these regulating mechanisms—the body's built-in thermostat—break down and are no longer able to do their job properly. If the core temperature rises above 38 degrees Centigrade or falls below 35 degrees Centigrade mental and physical control begin to fail. The victim quickly becomes unconscious and may die from heart or lung failure.

Climatic conditions to beware of

There are two weather combinations which are particularly dangerous:

Cold and Wet
and
Hot and Dry

Effects of excessive cold

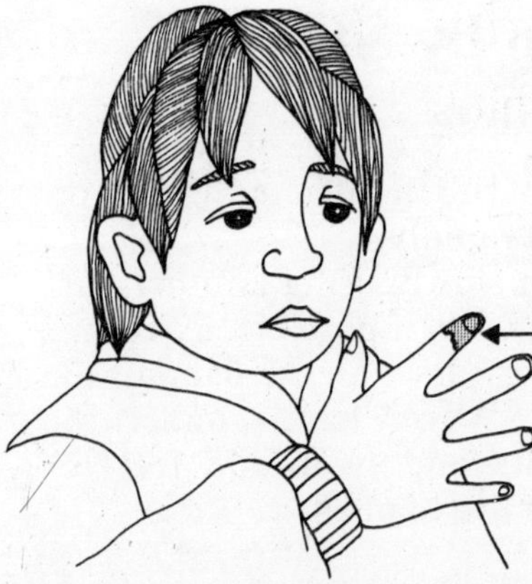

Frostbite: An exposed extremity—the nose, ears, fingers or toes—goes cold and very pale, becomes stiff and painful, turns numb and may eventually be paralysed.

Cold exhaustion: The victim is cold, wet and tired. As body temperature falls cold exhaustion sets in. Speech begins to slurr, the victim shivers and has cramps, his vision is disturbed and he begins to stumble.

Severe hypothermia: If the exposure continues, the body becomes very cold (25 degrees Centigrade) and breathing slows and becomes shallow. Eventually core temperature drops to 20 degrees Centigrade and the victim dies.

Groups liable to severe hypothermia

Mountaineering and hiking expeditions

Sailing parties—especially after capsizing

Old people without adequate home heating

Very young children who are not properly dressed and cared for

Drug addicts and alcoholics who sleep rough

Others who might undergo prolonged unconsciousness, e.g: diabetics and epileptics

Effects of excessive heat

Local burns: Prolonged exposure to the sun's ultra-violet rays can bring severe burns to any uncovered part of the body.

Heat exhaustion: In a hot climate heat is lost by evaporation of sweat from the skin. If this is excessive the body will run short of salt and water and this may be followed by vomiting and diarrhoea. Temperature usually remains close to normal, but the victim of heat exhaustion will be restless and complain of cramps.

Heat stroke: If the climate is hot and very humid little heat can be lost from the body by sweating. Core and surface temperatures therefore rise rapidly and this produces a headache and dizziness. The skin remains hot, dry and flushed and consciousness is rapidly lost.

Step by Step

Frostbite

Do not rub the affected area or reheat it rapidly.
Warm slowly using another part of the body if possible. Cover the nose or ears with the palm of the hand. Warm hands under the armpits and wrap the feet together in a blanket.

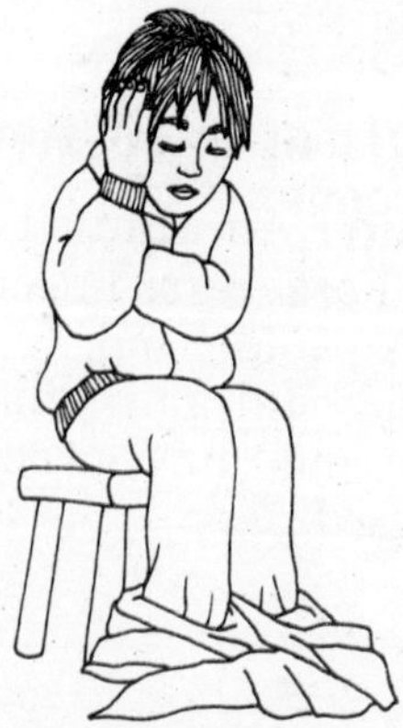

Frost bite and its first aid treatment

Cold exhaustion

Any expedition should be properly organised, planned and adequately supplied with wind and rain-proof clothing, shelter, energy-giving rations, flares, a large polythene bag, etc. Every member of the group should be fit and carry no more than one-third his own weight up to a maximum of 18 kilograms.

Severe hypothermia

If the victim of severe hypothermia is rewarmed rapidly, the blood vessels in the skin will dilate (enlarge) and draw blood supplies away from vital organs such as the brain. It is therefore essential that those suffering from severe hypothermia be reheated slowly by one or two blankets. Medical help should be urgently sought. If breathing or pulse stops, start immediate mouth to mouth resuscitation or external cardiac compression.

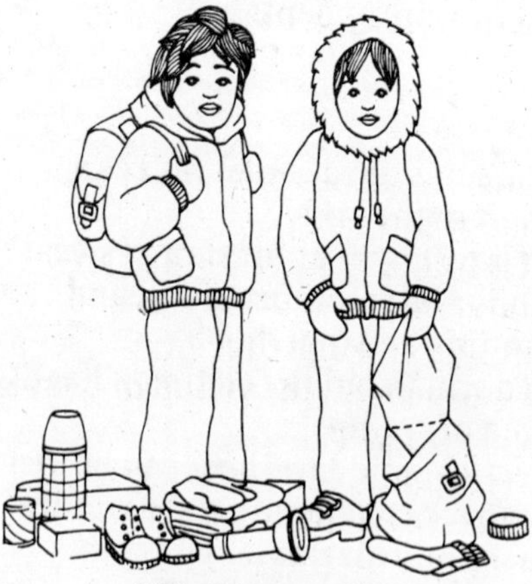

"Be Prepared"

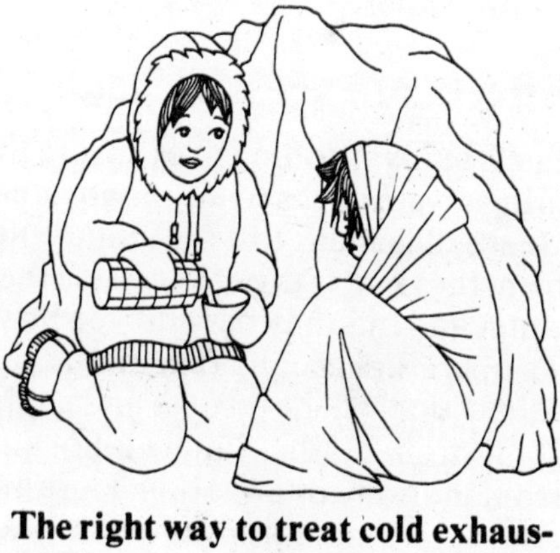

The right way to treat cold exhaustion

Do's

Rest: This is essential to overcoming exhaustion

Insulation: The victim should be wrapped up in a warm blanket or sleeping bag and his head covered over

Shelter: Atent or wind break such as a polythene sheet should be put up to reduce the victim's heat loss.

Food: If the victim is conscious he should be given warm, sweet drinks.

Rescue: Remove to base camp by the most comfortable method available.

At Base Camp: Reheat the victim rapidly by immersing the whole body in a hot bath (maximum temperature: 45 degrees Centigrade) Get medical help

Dont's

Do *not* apply hot water

Do *not* rub the skin

Do *not* give alcohol (each of these steps would produce increased skin blood flow and further reduce core temperature)

Local burns

See Chapter 2.

Heat exhaustion

Remove to the shade.

Add $\frac{1}{2}$ teaspoon of salt to a glass of water and feed to the victim. This will help replace the lost salt and fluids. Repeat the action but be careful not to administer too much salt as this will only make the victim ill and so aggravate the problem.

Heat stroke

The main aim here is to cool the victim. This should be done as follows:

- Remove to the shade
- Provide ventilation if possible (with a fan, etc.)
- Wrap in a damp sheet
- Seek medical help

Quiz

1) How is body temperature controlled?

2) What are the symptoms of cold exhaustion?

3) What groups of people are liable to cold exhaustion?

4) What is the difference between cold exhaustion and severe hypothermia?

5) How should severe hypothermia be treated?

6) What is the first-aid treatment for frostbite?

7) What is the difference between heat stroke and heat exhaustion?

8) How can the heat victim be cooled?

9) What is normal body temperature?

10) What preparations must be made before embarking on a long hike?

7 If breathing stops

You are at your local swimming baths. Suddenly, a young man starts struggling in the water and it is several minutes before he is pulled to safety. He looks terrible when you see him close up. His face and lips are blue. You put your ear to his chest and hear his heart beating weakly. Then you look at his mouth and realise that it is filled with frothy water. He has stopped breathing!

What would you do to save his life?

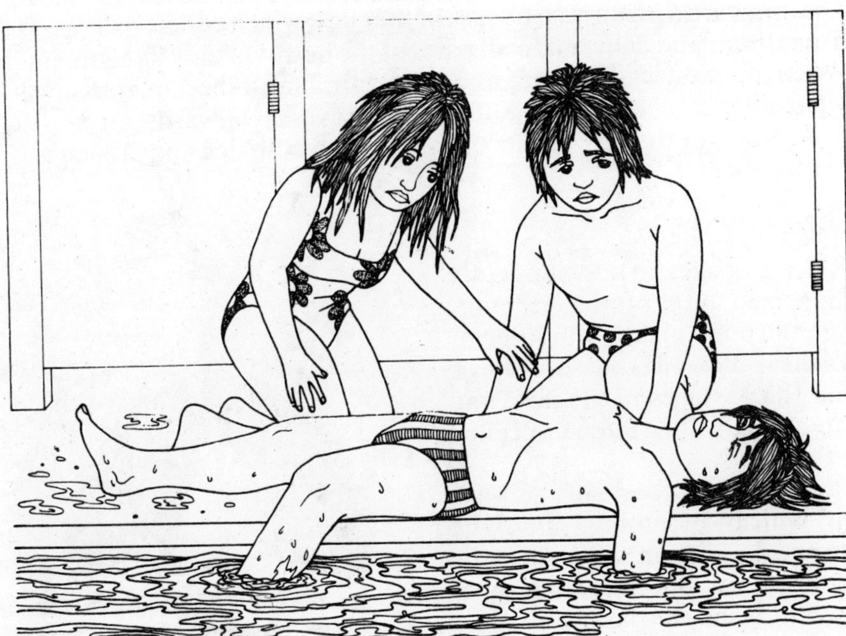

Theory

When someone stops breathing he is said to be asphyxiated or suffocated. This means the air is not reaching the lungs. Suffocation is one of the most important emergencies which the first aider must know about. Your action can save lives. In order to understand how to deal with a person who is not breathing, you must know a little about the body's breathing apparatus and how it works.

Air

The colourless, odourless atmosphere in which we live is called air and contains approximately 80 per cent nitrogen (N_2) and 20 per cent oxygen (O_2). Oxygen is essential to bodily processes so that if breathing stops, the individual will survive between only five and seven minutes—provided the heart continues to function. If the heart stops the survival time is reduced to a mere three minutes.

Breathing

The contraction of the diaphragm and the expansion of the chest wall act like bellows in the body sucking air into the lungs and pushing out unwanted carbon dioxide (CO_2). This constant inhaling and exhaling is called breathing.

Lungs

The lungs are a pair of elastic sacs in the chest which collect oxygen from the air and deliver it to all parts of the body via the bloodstream. When the chest wall expands and the diaphragm, a sheet of muscle separating the chest from the abdomen, moves downwards, air is pulled into the lungs: when it contracts carbon dioxide and other gases are expelled.

The airways

The air spaces in the lungs are connected to the atmosphere outside the body via the windpipe or trachea, the voice-box or larynx, and the passages in the nose and mouth. Together these are called the airways.

Drowning is just one of the ways in which breathing may be stopped. The airways may be blocked or the mechanism of breathing may be paralysed.

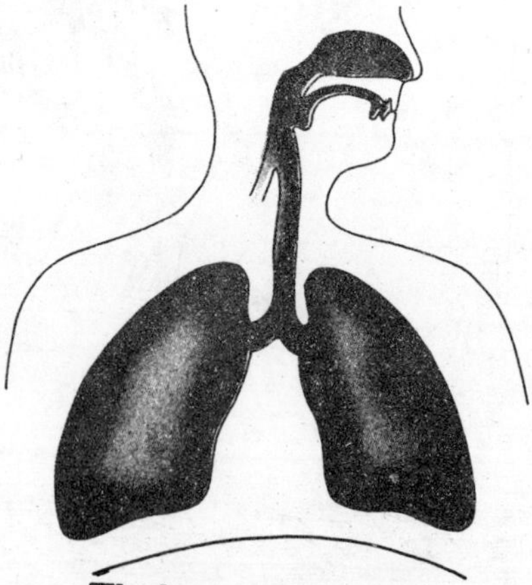

The lungs and airways

How breathing stops

Blocked airways: The airways may be blocked at any point. The most important sites are the pharynx (back of the mouth and nose) and the larynx. The pharynx may be blocked by the tongue, false teeth, vomit or blood. The larynx may be blocked by tight contraction of the vocal cords due to poisonous gases or inhaled material such as peanuts or fishbones.

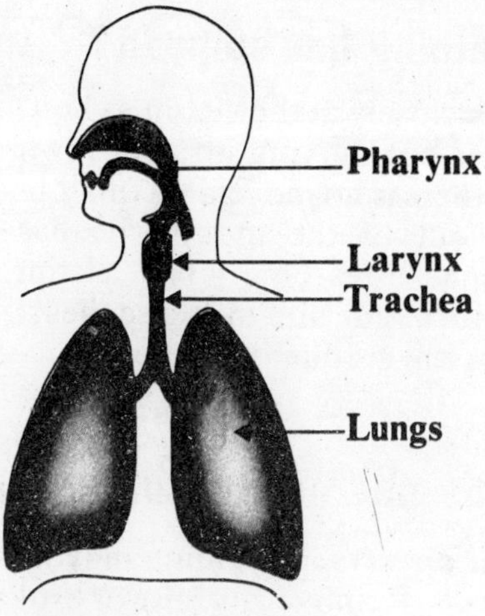

Obstruction

Paralysed breathing mechanism: The brain usually sends messages through the spinal cord and then the nerves to supply the muscles which move the chest wall and diaphragm. The brain may be damaged by an accident or a stroke, for example. The spinal cord may be injured by a broken neck, the nerves may be paralysed by poliomyelitis, or the chest wall may be unable to move because it is trapped by a heavy weight or because the ribs are badly broken. In any of these cases, breathing may be stopped.

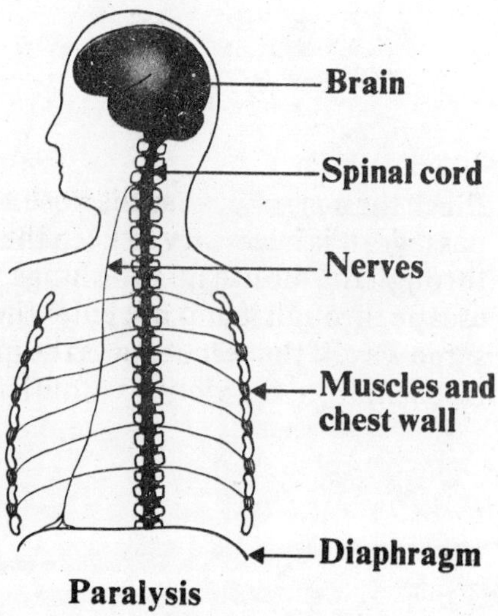

Paralysis

How do I know when breathing has stopped?

Look closely at the victim's chest. If it is not moving up and down and there is no movement of air in and out of the mouth, he has stopped breathing. The victim will turn blue and his pulse (heart beat) will gradually weaken.

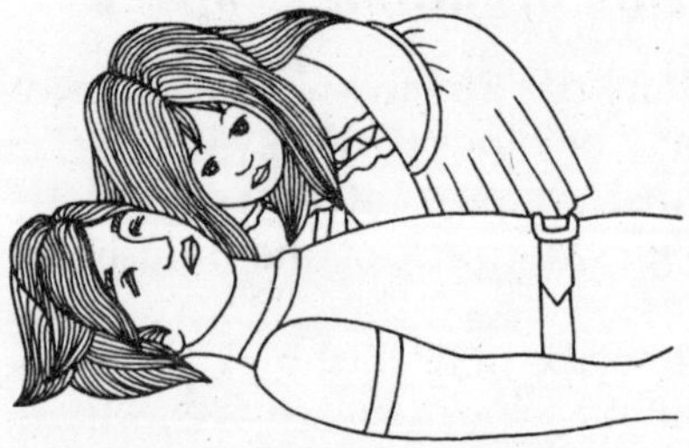

Has breathing stopped?

What emergency action should I take?

Clear airways: Breathing may be stopped by an obstruction in the airways. Remove any false or broken teeth, spit, phlegm, vomit, etc.

Extend neck and pull the jaw forward: When the victim is lying on his back with his head in the normal position, the tongue blocks the airways. Extending the neck and pulling the jaw forward keeps the top part of the airway open and allows air to pass through.

Pulling the head back stops the tongue blocking the airway

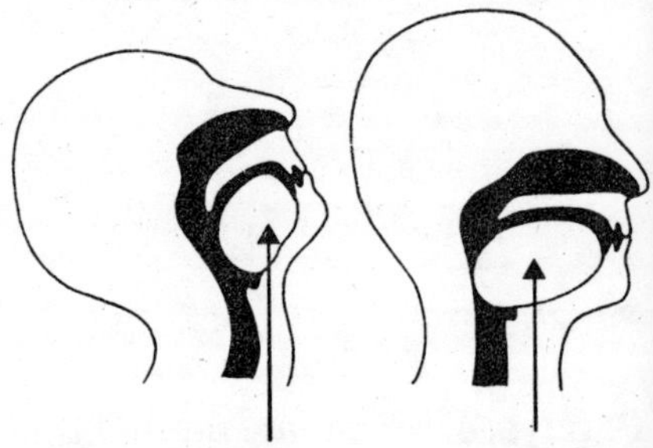

Airway open **Tongue blocks airway**

Pinch the nose: Because the nose and mouth are connected by an air passage, it is necessary to keep the nose closed when blowing air through the mouth into the lungs. If the nose were left open, air would escape through it and not enter the lungs where it is needed. In the same way, if the rescuer uses the mouth to nose method of resuscitation, the victim's mouth must be kept closed if it is to work.

Open the mouth and apply mouth to mouth resuscitation: The victim is now ready to have air blown into his lungs. Keep the neck extended and the jaw pulled forward, pinch the nose and apply your mouth to the victim's, forming an airtight seal.

Blow into the mouth—watch the chest. Does it rise?
If not, check the airways for obstructions (see page 55).

If it does rise, repeat the action two more times. This fills the lungs with air and gives you time to:

check that the pulse is strong
confirm that the victim is still not breathing

If the pulse is strong and he is *not* breathing, continue mouth to mouth resuscitation, inflating the chest about 15 times a minute.

Resuscitation should be continued until the victim begins breathing naturally again, or you are exhausted, or a doctor asks you to stop.

Step by Step

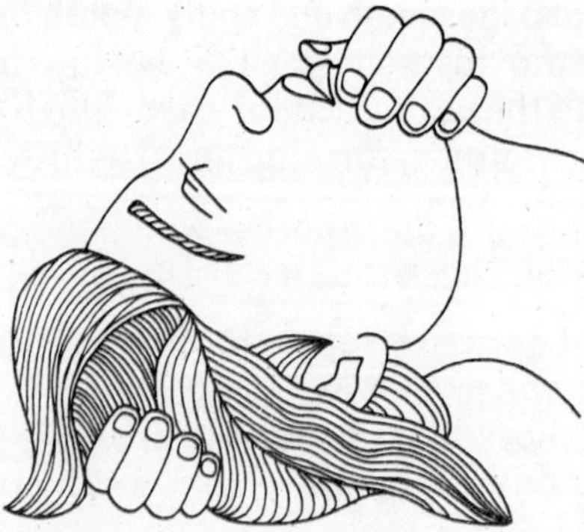

Extending the neck

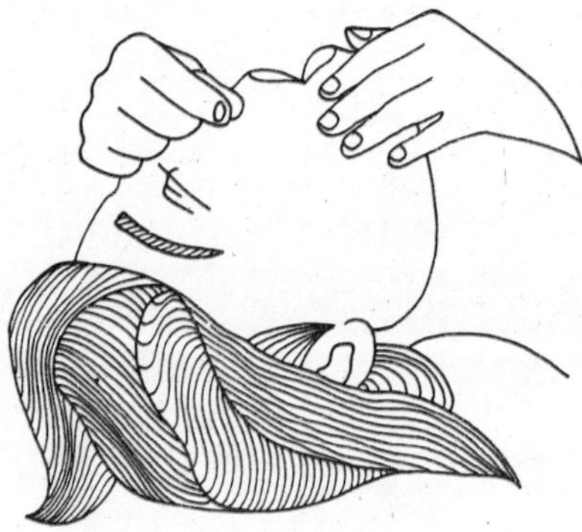

Pinching the nose and opening the mouth

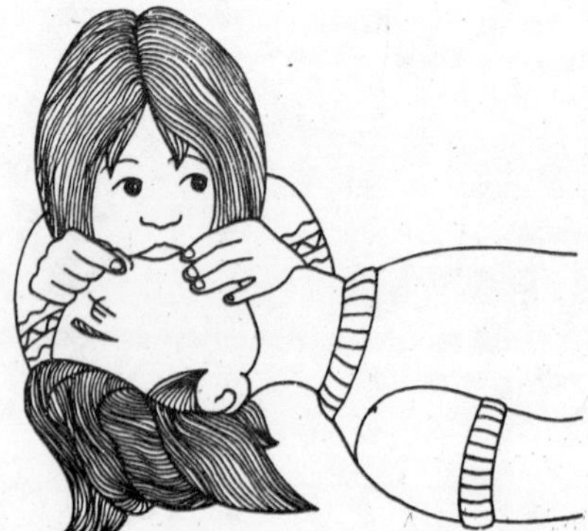

Mouth to mouth resuscitation

Blow into the mouth and watch the rise and fall of chest

Drowning

Begin resuscitation as soon as possible and keep the victim face up. (Turning the victim face down will not help empty water from the lungs.)

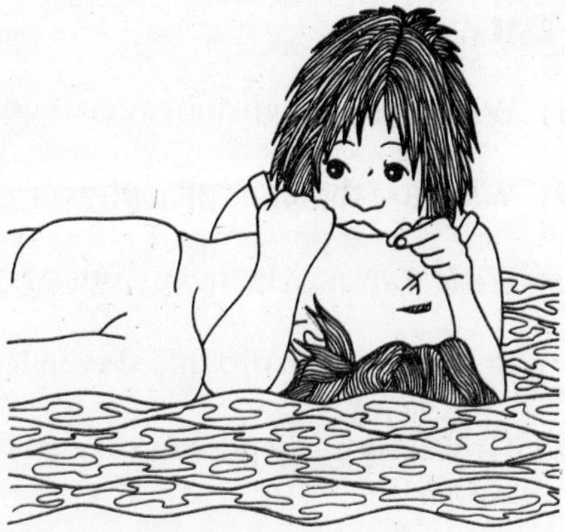

Electric shock

Switch off the current and pull the victim away from the source of the electricity. In cases of high voltage shock do not touch the victim, keep everyone else at least 20 metres away, and immediately inform the police by dialling 999 on the telephone. Only a small percentage of victims suffering from electric shocks will stop breathing. If this happens, mouth to mouth resuscitation should be started immediately. Burns, etc. should be dealt with only after spontaneous breathing has been restored.

Obstruction of airways

Produced by false teeth, a loose tooth, peanuts or some other material stuck in an airway, this usually results in violent efforts to breathe and is accompanied by a great deal of noise from the airways. Treatment is aimed at dislodging the foreign body. A child should be turned upside down and shaken until the foreign body is removed. An adult should be bent over the knee and hit on the back until the obstruction has cleared away.

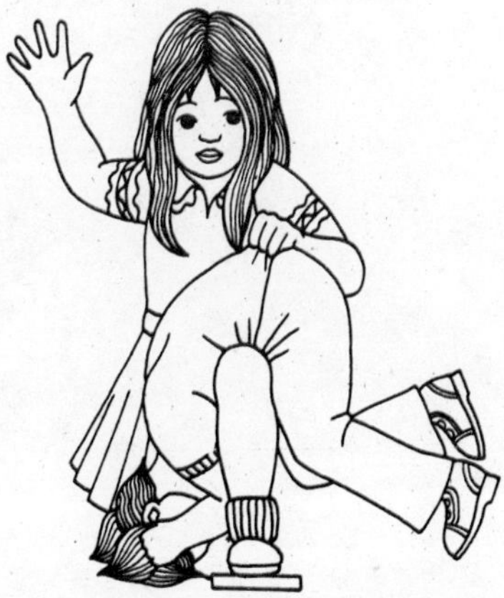

Quiz

1) What percentage of oxygen is contained in air?

2) What are the signs of asphyxia?

3) How is air moved in and out of the lungs?

4) Should carbon dioxide stay in the lungs?

5) How long can a person survive without oxygen after breathing stops?

6) Why is it necessary to extend the neck and pull the jaw forward?

7) How many times a minute should you blow into the chest during mouth to mouth resuscitation?

8) What is the first thing you must do to someone suffering from electric shock?

9) How would you clear an obstruction from the airways of an adult?

10) Why pinch the nose during mouth to mouth resuscitation?

8 How to control bleeding

On a camping holiday you see a young man chopping up wood. You watch fascinated as his blows transform a large log into bits small enough to fuel a camp fire. Then in a flash the axe bounces off the wood and cuts deep into the chopper's leg. Blood begins gushing from the wound and he staggers to the ground. He goes into a cold sweat, turns deathly white and faints. His breathing becomes shallow and you quickly check his pulse. It is beating rapidly but becoming weaker.

What would you do to save his life?

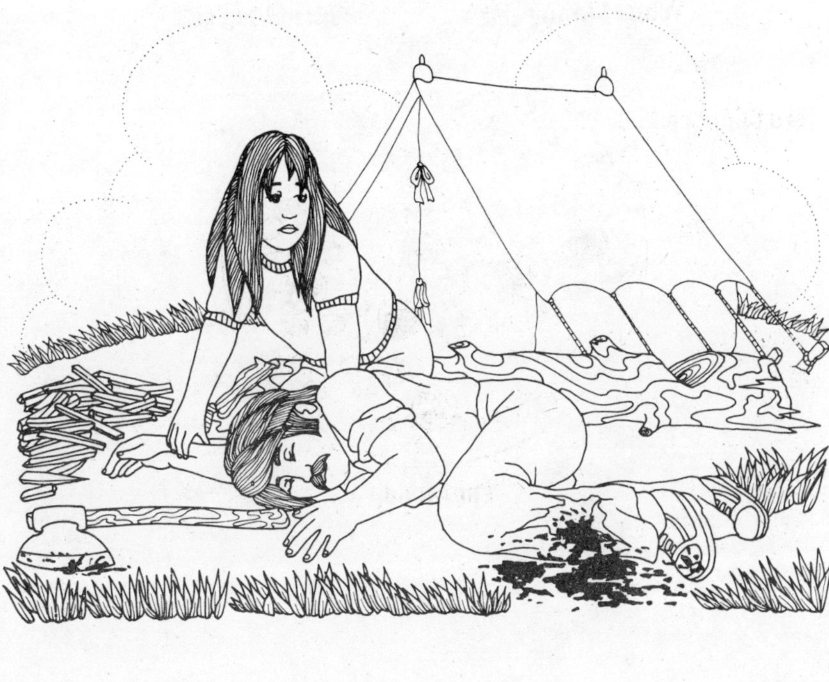

Theory

Blood

Blood is an important biological fluid which circulates constantly through the heart, lungs and body. A full-grown person has approximately five litres of blood in his body. If more than one litre of this is lost (or proportionately less in a child), the person's life is in great danger and the bleeding must be stopped and the victim taken to the nearest hospital for a transfusion.

Blood is made up of the following main parts:

Red blood cells which contain the red pigment haemoglobin. This substance is responsible for carrying oxygen around the body.

White blood cells which protect the body from infection. Pus is largely made up from these cells.

Plasma which is a straw-coloured thick liquid in which blood cells are suspended and food stuffs dissolved.

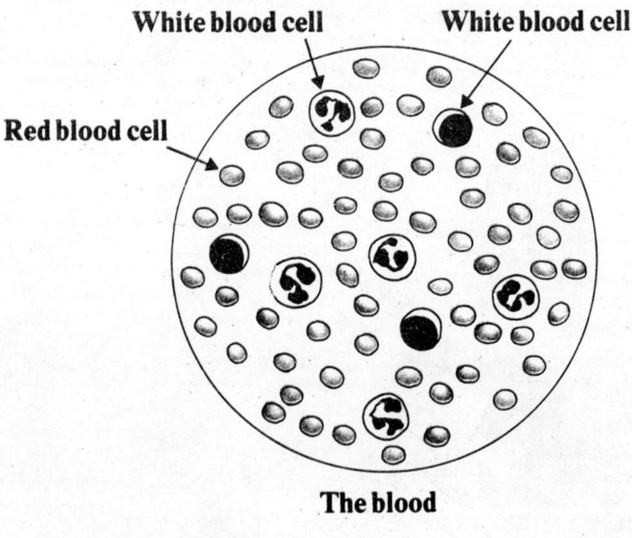

The blood

Bleeding

The arteries which lead from the heart are strong muscular and elastic tubes which contain blood under high pressure. Veins which go to the heart contain blood at low pressure. Between the arteries and veins are many microscopic tubes called capillaries. Bleeding can occur from any of these three types of vessels.

Each type of vessel bleeds in a different way:

Arterial bleeding occurs in spurts of blood in time with the heart beat.

Venous bleeding is a strong, steady flow.

Capillary bleeding is a slow, steady flow which quickly stops.

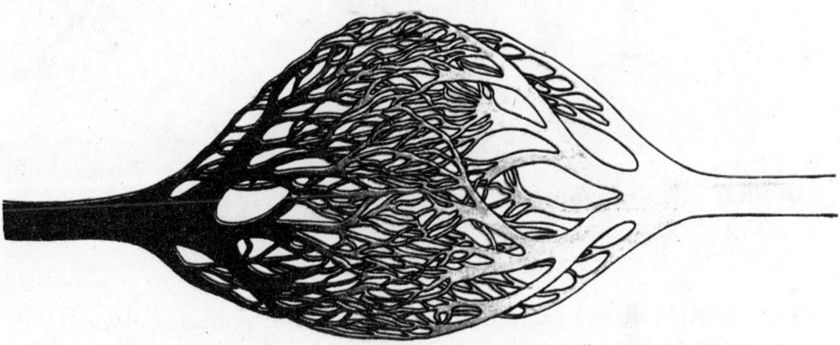

How the body stops bleeding

When the skin is cut blood vessels are severed and bleeding follows. When this happens the blood vessels tighten up or contract, blood clots, and if much blood is lost, blood pressure falls. In these three ways blood loss is reduced.

Finding the pulses and pressure points

Each time the heart beats the blood pressure increases and a 'pulse' can be felt in the arteries. This pulse can be taken best where the artery can be pressed against a bone (at the pressure points).

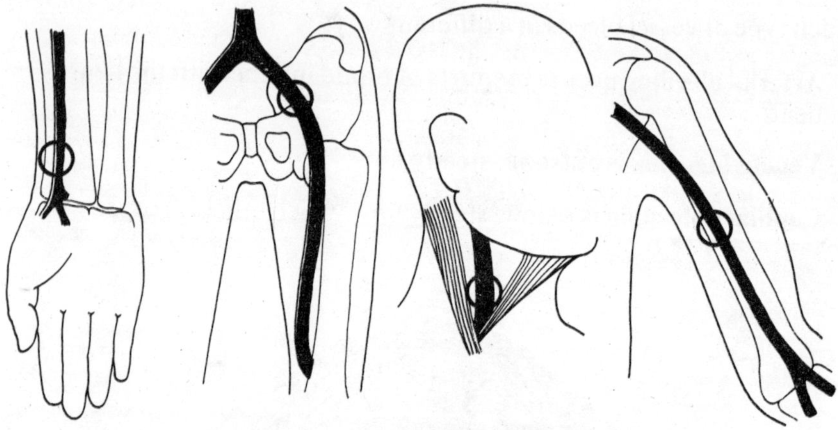

Radial **Femoral** **Carotid** **Brachial**

Neck or carotid pulse: Located at the point of the triangle between the shaded muscle which runs from the ear to the collar bone and the muscles covering the voice box (larynx) and the windpipe (trachea).

Wrist or radial pulse: Can be found at the thumb side of the wrist in the position where the watch strap is usually worn. This is not a pressure point because the hand is also supplied by another artery.

Arm or brachial pulse: Felt halfway down the inside of the arm between the bands of muscles above and below the arm bone. A nerve runs ng this artery and if it is rolled on the bone it will produce a tingling ·ion in the arm and little finger.

..igh or fermoral pulse: Positioned halfway between the centre of the pubic bone and the front of the hip bone. This point is just on the inside of the leg below the groin skin crease.

When light pressure is applied to the artery, the pulse can be felt and counted, and have its strength measured. The normal pulse is between 60 to 90 beats a minute and should feel full and strong. Locate the pulses on yourself and practise how to find them quickly.
If heavy pressure is applied to these sites, the arteries will be pushed against the bone and no blood will flow through. This may be used to control bleeding in a site supplied by that particular artery.

Internal bleeding

Several important organs such as the liver, spleen and kidneys are protected by the lower ribs. If these are broken the jagged ends of the ribs may puncture the tissues and cause serious internal bleeding. Broken bones and other damaged organs may also bleed.
Often the only external signs of internal bleeding may be the development of shock (see signs of shock below) and/or the following:

Vomiting or coughing up blood
Passing blood in the urine
Swelling of a limb around a broken bone
Bruising over the lower ribs

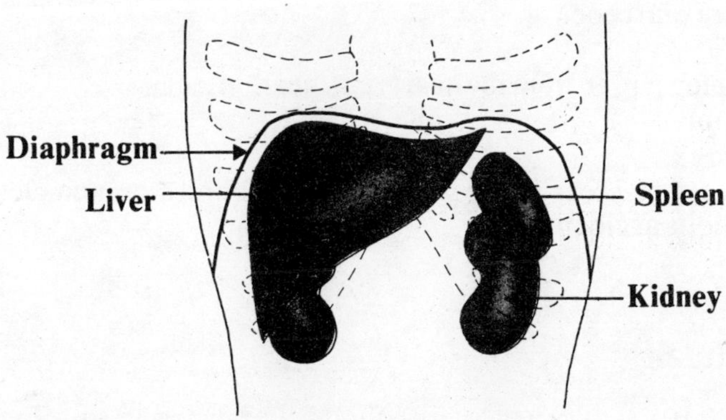

External bleeding

This may happen if the skin is lacerated (torn with ragged edges), incised (cut with smooth edges like a razor slash), or stabbed. There would have to be a severe loss of blood before the victim's life was endangered, but even a little blood can look a lot if you are not used to dealing with it. The First-Aider is in a good position to deal with any of these and to control or stop external bleeding.

What is shock ?

When the blood does not circulate properly to the tissues, they become deprived of oxygen and other essential foodstuffs. The victim is then said to be 'shocked' or 'in shock'.
This poor circulation of blood may be due to:

Loss of blood: e.g. internal bleeding
external bleeding

Loss of fluid: e.g. from burns
from severe vomiting
from severe diarrhoea

Loss of pumping power from the heart: e.g. heart attacks
heart failure

Following a very severe fright or severe pain: e.g. burst stomach ulcer
after a serious accident

ABC of shock

It is important to be able to recognise shock. The victim in shock may show any or all of the following signs:

Anxious and trembling
Blueness of the lips and paleness of the skin
Cold clammy skin
Dryness of the mouth
Eyesight blurred and concentration poor
Fast pulse

A victim in shock needs careful treatment:

- Tight clothing should be loosened and crowds should be moved away to allow the injured person to breath and relieve his anxiety.
- The victim must be laid flat to improve circulation to the brain.
- The legs should be raised to draw all available blood into the important part of the body and improve the circulation.

Shock occasionally produces difficulty in breathing. If this happens prop the victim up. The victim in shock should never be given anything to drink (water or alcohol, etc.) because an emergency operation may be necessary.

Fainting

This is a temporary and very mild form of poor blood circulation to the brain. The person who has fainted usually falls to the ground, sweats, and has a fast pulse. Nothing needs to be done except perhaps to loosen tight clothing and to raise the legs. The victim will recover rapidly on his own.

A dirty wound

A wound is a breach in the protective layer covering the body. Germs such as bacteria and viruses enter the body through it and cause infections. This risk of serious complications is much greater when the wound is dirty or left open to the air. Dirty wounds should be washed with clean water or with a dilute solution of antiseptic, dressed and bandaged. A doctor should see any victim with a dirty wound because antibiotic and anti-tetanus injections may be needed.

Step by Step

External bleeding

Lie the victim down.
Loosen tight clothing and expose the bleeding part.
Apply direct pressure to the wound using:

Dressings
Bandages
Clean handkerchiefs
Tissues
Fresh newspapers, etc.

Raise the wounded part to lower the blood pressure in this area.
Bandage the dressings in place.
If bleeding does not stop apply more dressings. If this is not sufficient apply pressure to the Pressure (pulse) Point for a maximum of 15 minutes. Pressure can be re-applied after allowing one minute for the circulation to reach the limb. Arrange medical help as necessary. Check for pulse and general condition.

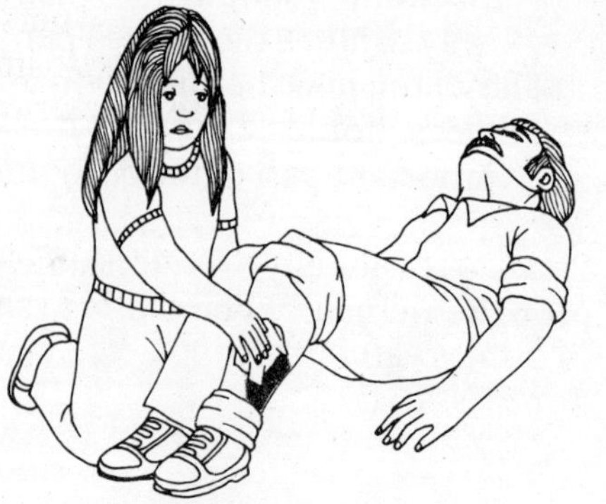

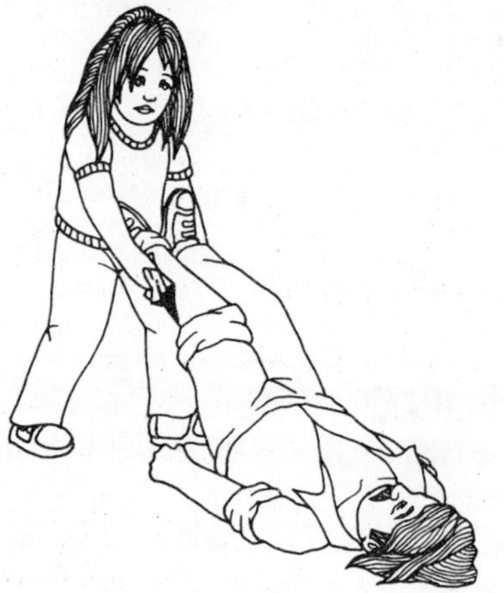

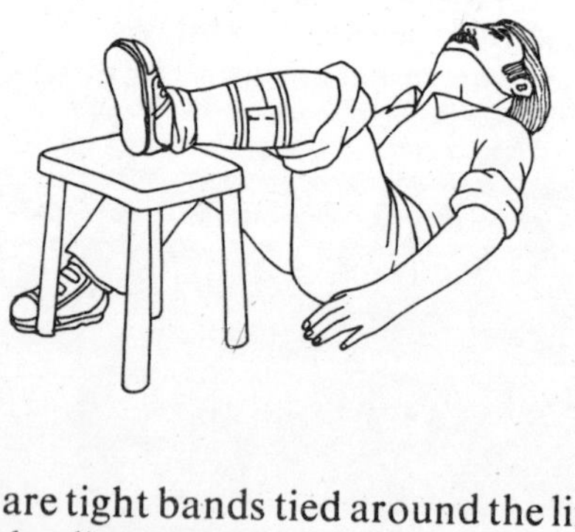

Tourniquets: These are tight bands tied around the limb often used in the past to prevent bleeding (see illustration page 8) but it is no longer recommended because it also restricts the return of blood to the heart through the veins and, if left in place for more than 15 minutes, may cause limbs to become gangrenous (dead).

Internal bleeding

Lie the victim down, loosen tight clothing, raise the legs and check his general condition. Get medical help as quickly as possible and try to comfort him.

Ear canal

Bleeding from the ear canal may be produced by a serious skull injury or by poking the ear. The First-Aider should do nothing other than cover the ear with a pad to reduce infection and get medical help quickly.

Nose

When hit or picked the nose usually bleeds and this is best treated by direct pressure. Pinch the nose between your finger and thumb. Sit the victim forward with his head over a sink—about ten minutes should be sufficient.

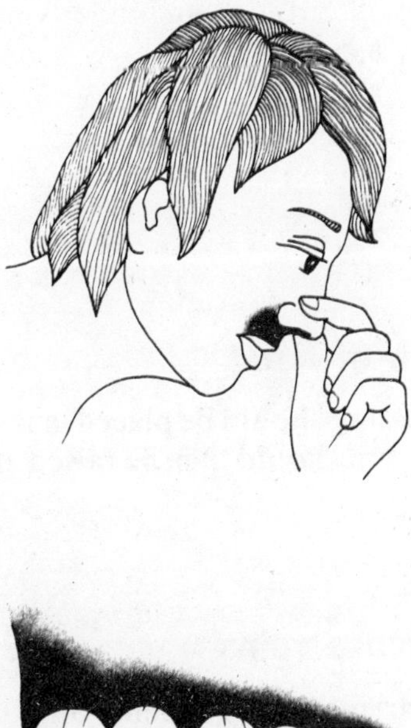

Gum

A bleeding tooth socket may be treated by placing a wad of cotton wool, tissues or handkerchief over the bleeding area, but not in the tooth socket, and having the victim bite down on the dressing. After ten minutes the bleeding will usually have stopped and the dressing can be removed. The victim should then sit upright and should neither walk about nor lie down.

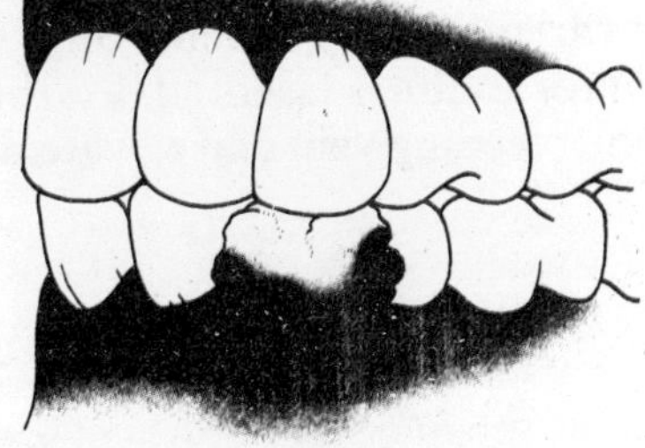

Lip, tongue or cheek

The bleeding part should be grasped between a dressing and local pressure applied for approximately ten minutes.

Scalp

When the scalp is wounded there is always the possibility that the skull underneath is broken. For this reason it is advisable not to apply direct pressure but place a ring pad on the wound instead. This will protect an underlying fracture.

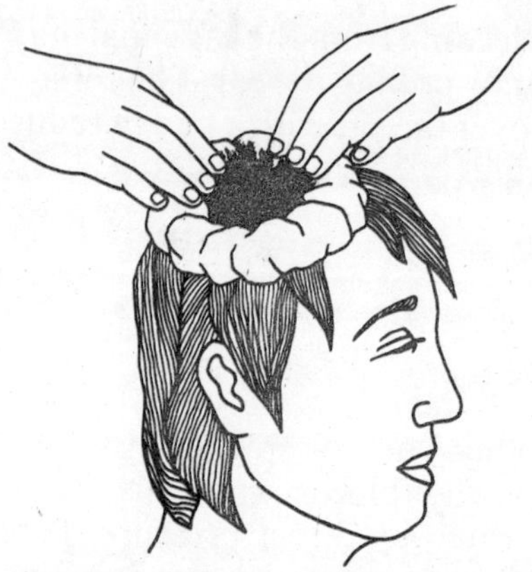

Palm of hand

A dressing should be placed in the palm and the hand closed tightly. The hand should then be raised and supported in a sling.

Varicose veins

If a varicose vein suddenly bursts the loss of blood may be torrential. Prompt action is essential. Lie the victim down, apply direct pressure to the bleeding vein and elevate the leg.

Foreign bodies in the wound

Where a foreign body such as glass or a fish hook remains in a bleeding wound, it should be removed only if it can be done easily. If the foreign body is stuck leave it in position. No direct pressure can be applied in this case and a ring pad must be used.

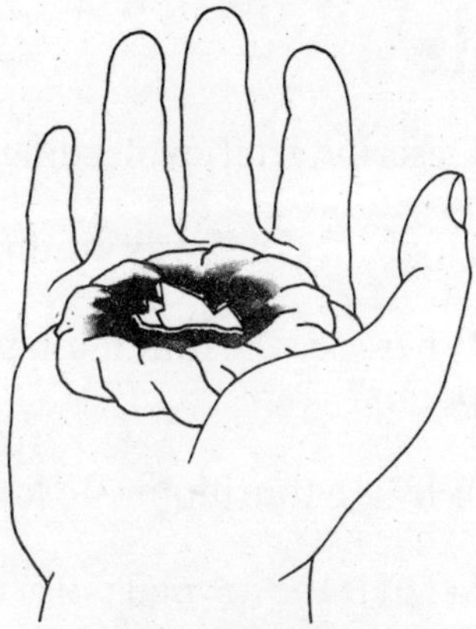

Bruises

These are often called contusions and are a form of internal bleeding just under the skin (a black eye is one example). There is rarely very serious bleeding and contusions should be treated with a cold compress or ice pack.

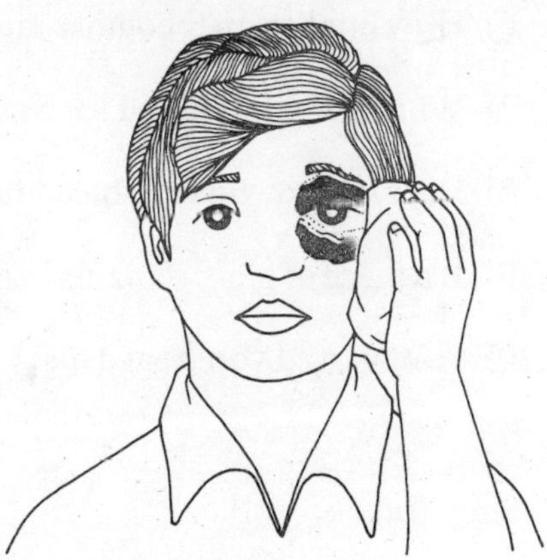

Penetrating wound

Chest: A stab wound in the chest may cause serious internal bleeding which will require urgent hospital treatment. It may also collapse the lung by allowing air to enter the space between the lung and the chest wall. This may partially be prevented by applying a dressing over the wound.

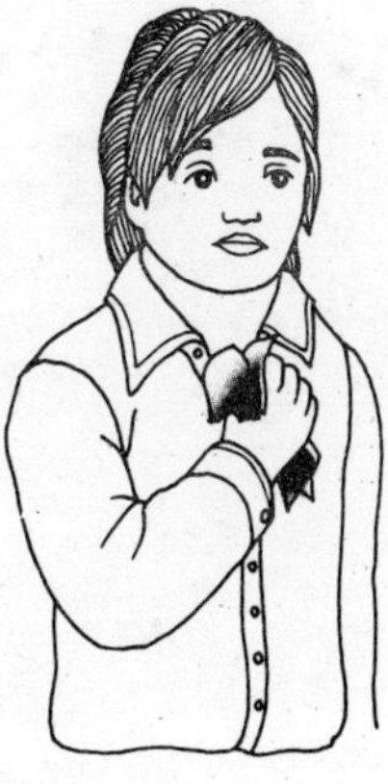

Abdomen: This may also result in severe internal bleeding or cause serious damage to an internal organ. Medical help must be sought urgently.

Quiz

1) Describe arterial bleeding.
2) How does the body minimise blood loss?
3) Where are the four main pulses and which of these are pressure points?
4) Why is a tourniquet no longer used to control bleeding?
5) What is the normal pulse rate?
6) How might you recognise internal bleeding?
7) What is the treatment for a nose bleed?
8) How would you stop bleeding in the gums?
9) If a piece of glass remains in a wound should it be removed?
10) How would you treat a black eye?

9 When the heart stops

You are returning from a football match. As you pass an elderly neighbour's house he stands up to greet you and, without warning, cries out in pain and slumps to the ground. He had been suffering from severe pains in the chest recently and was told by his doctor not to do any heavy work as these pains were from his heart. But the old man did not consider gardening "hard work" and so spent the day digging and planting in the warm sunshine. Now, he is lying unconscious on the grass. His lips and fingers are turning blue and he is breathing heavily. You listen to his chest but cannot hear the customary beating. His heart has stopped!

What would you do to save his life?

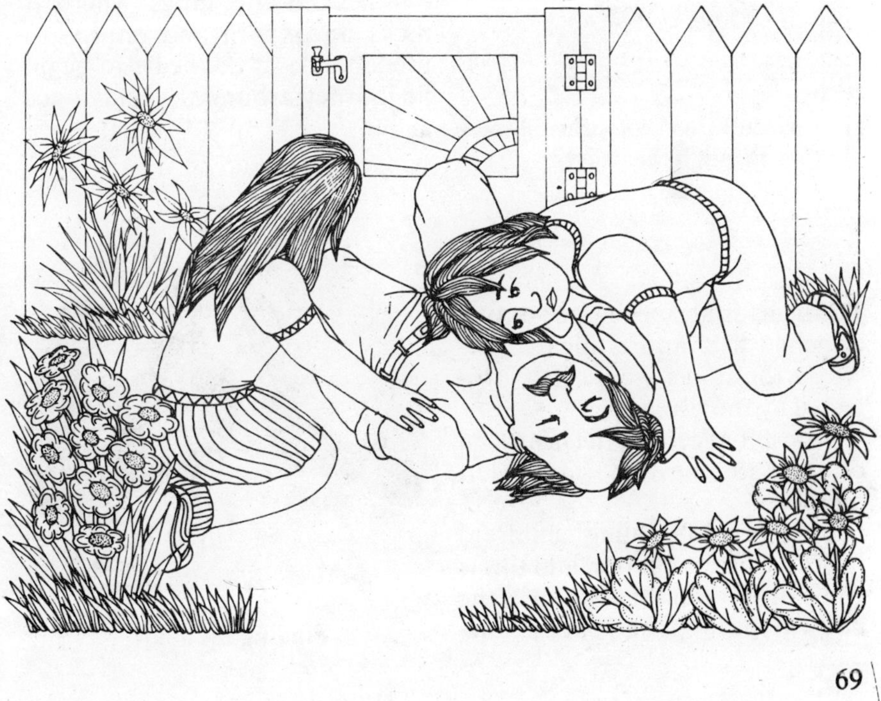

Theory

The heart is a muscular pump which circulates blood around the body. It is made up of two similar pumps which work side by side. The one on the right accepts blood from the body and circulates it to the lungs. The pump on the left then pushes the blood around the body.

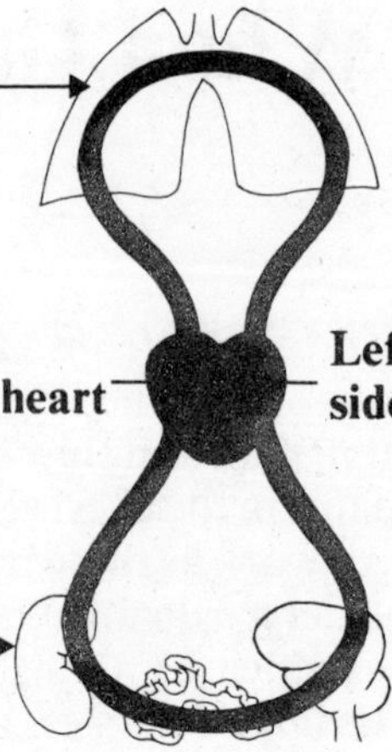

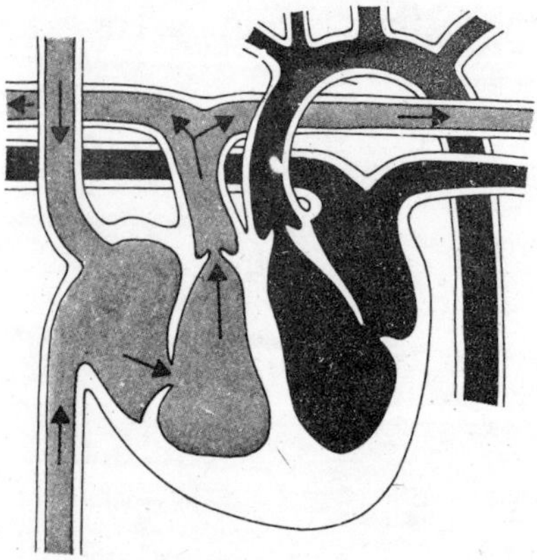

The circulation of the blood through the heart

The heart contains valves which make sure the blood travels only in one direction. As the blood circulates around the body, oxygen is removed, and the blood is carried back to the right side of the heart by the veins. It is then pumped to the lungs where it picks up oxygen and returns to the left side of the heart to begin its journey around the body once again.

The heart is about the size of two clenched fists and is located between the lungs where it is protected by the rib cage.

A little left of centre, the heart can often be seen beating near the left nipple.

People (except young children) have five litres of blood and this is constantly pumped from the body to the lungs and back again.

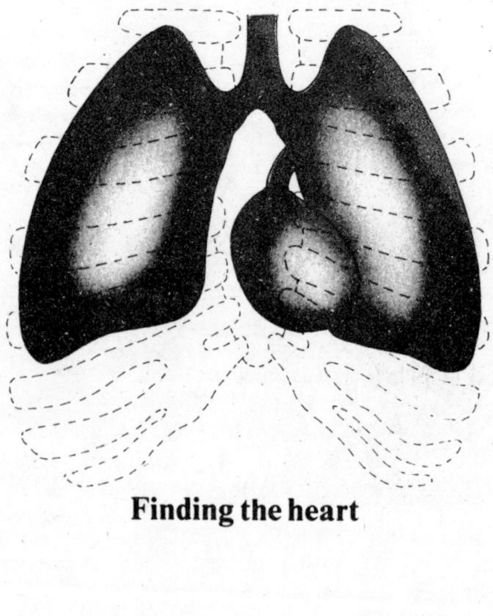

Finding the heart

When does the heart stop?

When the heart stops the victim is said to have a 'cardiac arrest'. This can be caused by:

When breathing stops ('ventilatory arrest')
Following strokes
Poisoning
Electric shock
Heart attack
Severe injury

Feel the carotid pulse

Within a few seconds of the heart stopping the victim loses consciousness and the skin looses its colour and becomes white often with a tinge of blue around the lips. The pulse may slow down until at last it disappears completely, or stop abruptly. The

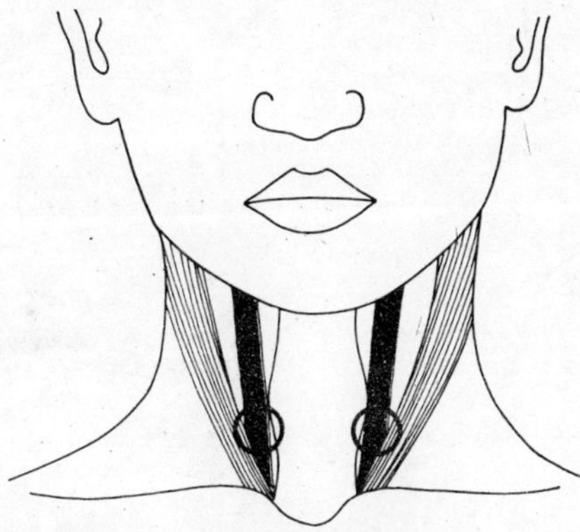

The carotid pulse

pupils widen. In cases of suspected cardiac arrest check the neck or carotid pulse to see if the heart is still beating. This pulse can be felt in the triangle between the windpipe and the shaded muscle which runs between the bone beneath the ear and the collar bone. Do not use the wrist pulse because it may be difficult to find and if it is weak it cannot be felt even though the heart is still beating. If the heart does not restart the victim will soon stop breathing and the brain will be permanently damaged by the lack of blood supply in about three minutes. It is therefore vital that the heart quickly begins pumping again or that the blood keeps flowing to the brain. Only the person on the spot can do this within the time limit and the First Aider is in a unique position to save a life in such a situation by external cardiac compression.

External cardiac compression

External cardiac compression is the name given to the artificial way of keeping the blood circulating to the vital organs and particularly the brain. The heart lies between the breast bone (sternum) at the front of the body and the back bone (vertebral column) at the back. Lie the victim face up on a hard surface like the floor and not a soft bed. This will keep the victim rigid. The breast bone can then be pressed down towards the backbone. The heart will be compressed and blood squeezed out into the circulatory system.

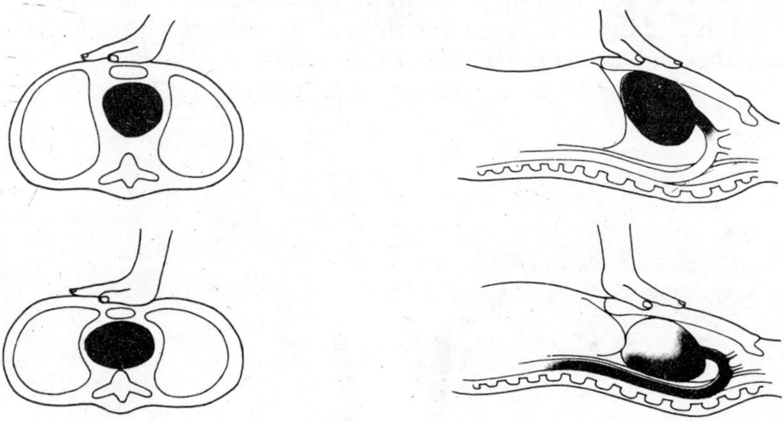

External cardiac compression with mouth to mouth resuscitation

When the heart stops the brain is deprived of oxygen with the result that the part of the brain which controls breathing quickly stops working and the victim stops breathing. Likewise if the victim stops breathing, the heart will not receive oxygen and will not beat properly. If these two situations occur at the same time both external cardiac compression and mouth to mouth resuscitation will be needed to save the victim.

If two people are available then one should concentrate on giving mouth to mouth resuscitation, checking the pupil size (are they wide or narrow?), and feeling the neck pulse. The other should carry on with the external cardiac compression. It is important that the chest should not be inflated at the same time as the heart is compressed. A rhythm of one inflation of the chest followed by five external cardiac compressions repeated ten times a minute produces the best results. If only one person is available to give first aid many precious minutes can be wasted by switching from external cardiac compression to giving mouth to mouth resuscitation. The best method is to inflate the chest twice and then compress the heart 15 times. This should be done at the rate of four times a minute.

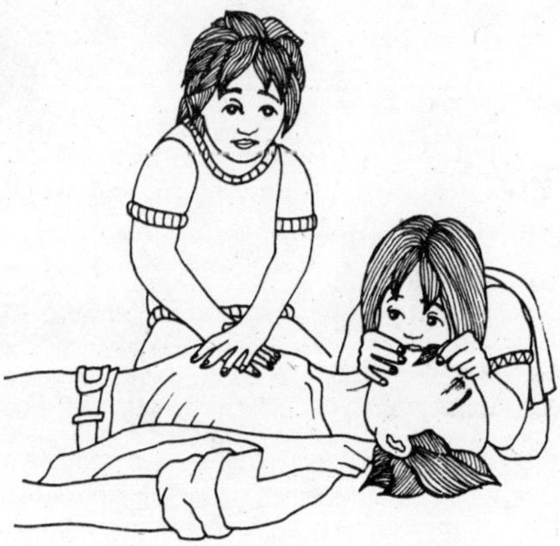

	One person	Two persons
Lungs	Two chest inflations	One chest inflation
	followed by	followed by
Heart	15 cardiac compressions	5 cardiac compressions
	repeated	repeated
Frequency	4 times a minute	10 times a minute

Step by Step

Feel the carotid pulse

This will confirm that the heart has stopped. Quickly place the victim on a hard surface and kneel beside him.

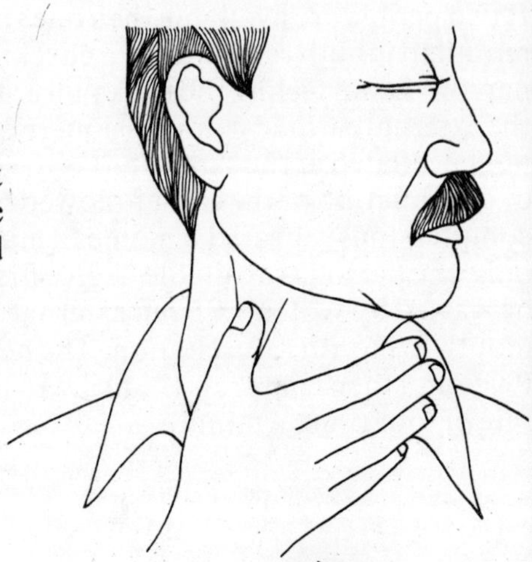

Strike the lower breastbone sharply

This should be done with the side of the hand. It may shock the heart into restarting. Feel the pulse. If the heart is not beating then start external cardiac compression.

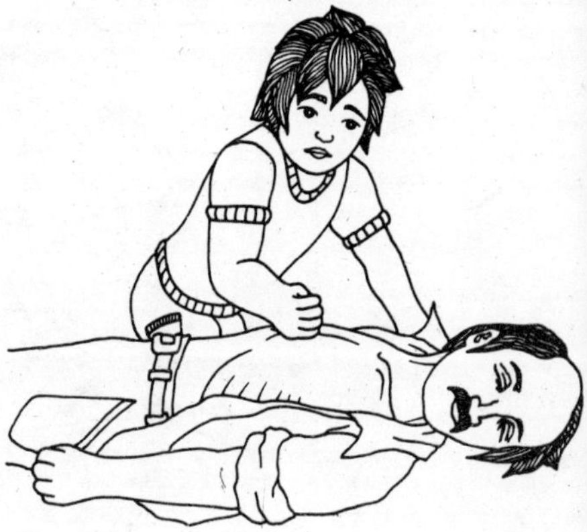

Compress the heart

Place the heel of the hand two-thirds of the way down the breastbone and press downwards. Considerable pressure is needed because the breastbone must be moved about four to five centimetres each time. This should be repeated about 60 times a minute.

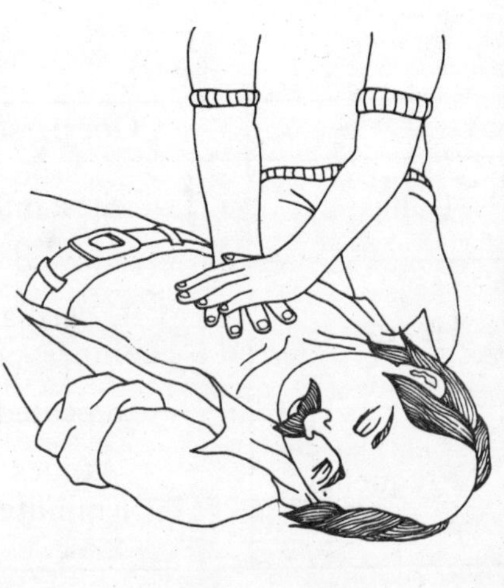

How do I know the heart's working

the pupils in the eye will become smaller
some colour will return to the face
a strong carotid pulse will be felt with each compression

How long do I carry on

until the heart starts beating by itself again

OR

an ambulance man, nurse or doctor, or more experienced first-aider tells you to stop

OR

you feel completely worn out

The victim is not dead until *you* have given up trying to resuscitate him.

External cardiac compression in babies and young children

The hearts of infants are much smaller than adults and must be compressed with less force. For instance, a baby of less than one year old needs about 120 compressions each minute. But it takes very little force to move a baby's breastbone and one thumb is all that is needed to produce the necessary pressure. It is also important to realise that an infant's heart is much higher in the chest and that the breast bone must be pressed in the middle and not over the lower half.

	Adult	Child	Infant
How far	5 cm.	2–4 cm.	1–2 cm.
How often	60	90	120
Where	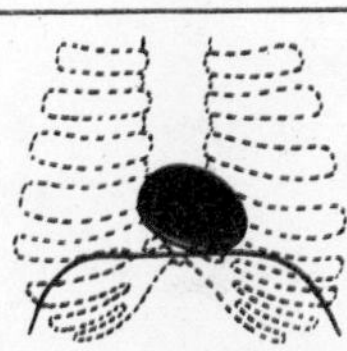	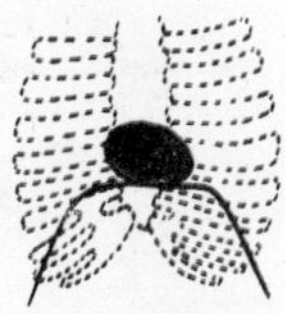	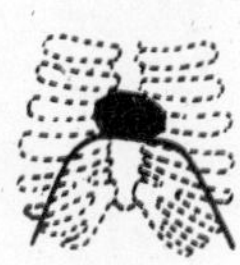
How	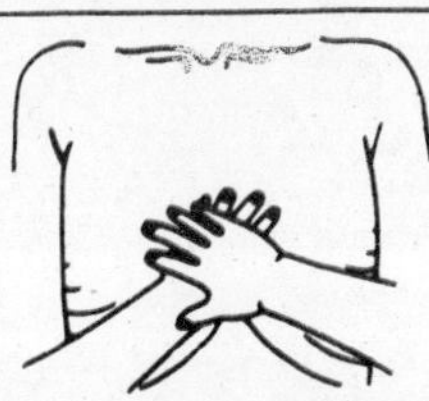	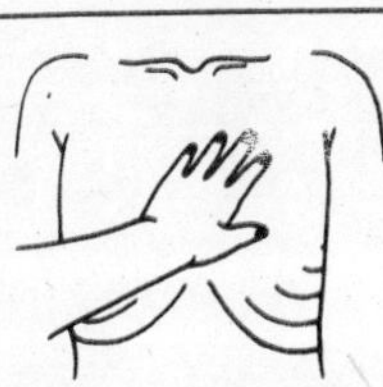	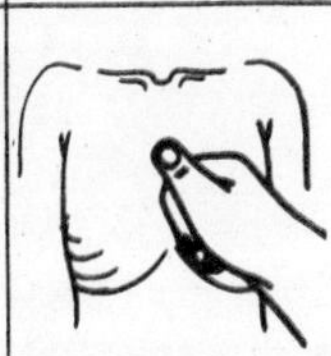

Quiz

1) To where is the blood pumped from the right hand side of the heart?

2) What is the size of the heart and where is it found?

3) How do you find the carotid pulse?

4) What are the causes of cardiac arrest?

5) Describe external cardiac compression.

6) When does permanent damage follow cardiac arrest?

7) If an adult's heart stops how many cardiac compressions should be performed each minute?

8) If you are the only person on the scene and a victim needs mouth to mouth resuscitation and external cardiac compression, how many should you apply of each and how often?

9) What are the differences in external cardiac compression between adults and young children?

10) How would you check that the heart is pumping properly again?

10 Just an ache or pain?

You go into a café for some coffee. While waiting for the waitress to take your order the woman at the next table is served fish and chips. A few minutes later you notice that she is coughing violently and turn around to see what is happening. She has a look of panic and her face is going blue. One of the bones in her fish is stuck in her throat and is choking her.

What would you do to save her life?

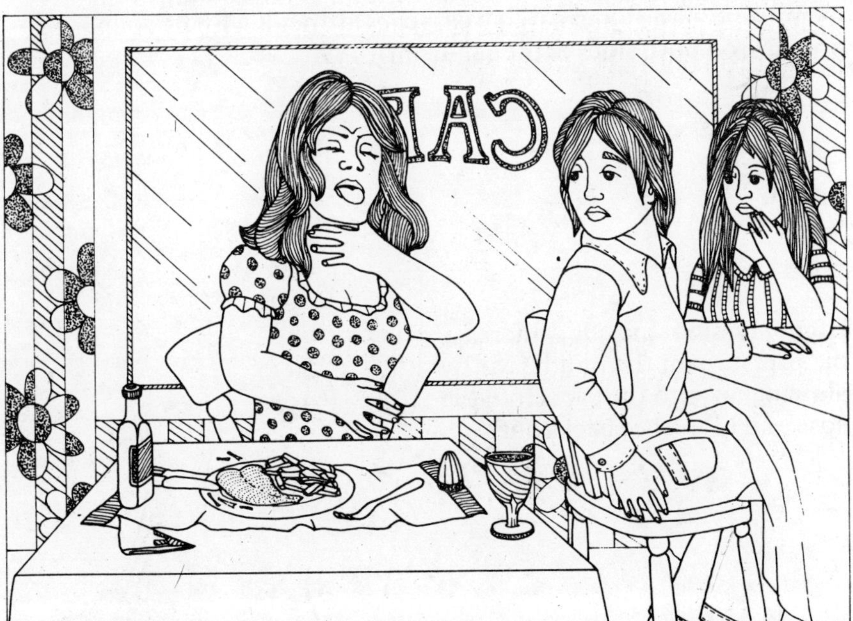

First-Aiders are often asked to help with aches and pains. Caused by heat, cold, pressure, stretching or sharp movements, most pains are not serious but it is always useful to be able to help relieve suffering and comfort the victim. If qualified medical help is not available the conditions described below can usually be temporarily eased by pain-relieving drugs, but taking these is always the responsibility of the victim. One tablet of paracetamol every two hours is a safe form of treatment.

Toothache

Treatment for toothache is simple: rest, avoid the extremes of hot and cold, keep the mouth warm and go to the dentist or doctor.

Earache

This is produced by pressure which stretches part of the inner ear. It can be caused by high pressure—for example, when diving and swimming under water or coming into land in aeroplane: low pressure (i.e. taking off in an aeroplane) can also cause some pain in the ear. Inflammation of the ear can also cause painful stretching of the membrane in the inner ear. All earaches are dealt with by equalising pressure on both sides of the ear drum.

High pressure outside: Increase the pressure on the middle ear by blowing air into the ear. Hold the nose and blow the cheeks out.

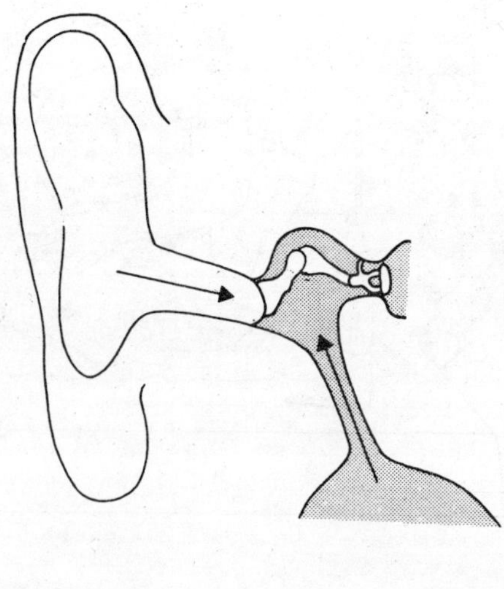

Low pressure outside: Lessen the pressure on the middle ear by swallowing.

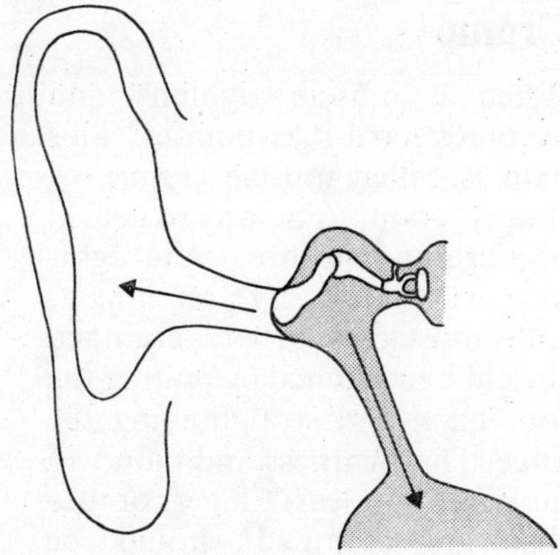

Pressure increase caused by inflammation: In this case pressure cannot be reduced because the tube leading from the inside of the ear to the back of the throat is blocked. Take the victim to the doctor.

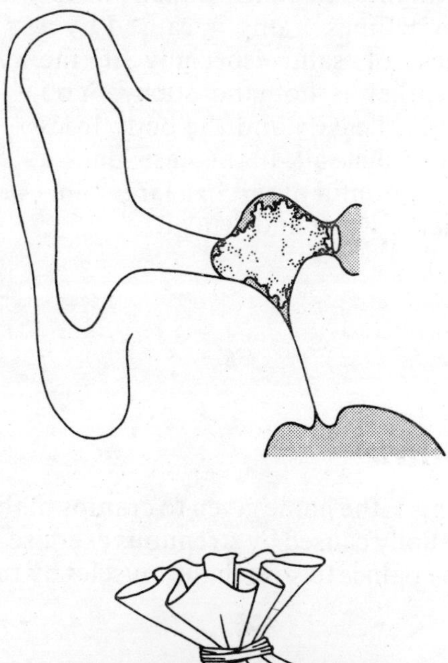

Black eye

If someone is hit in the eye bruising (light bleeding into the tissues) and swelling will develop. The bleeding stretches the tissues and causes pain. Swelling can be reduced by applying an ice-pack to the eye. As swelling goes down the pain is lessened.

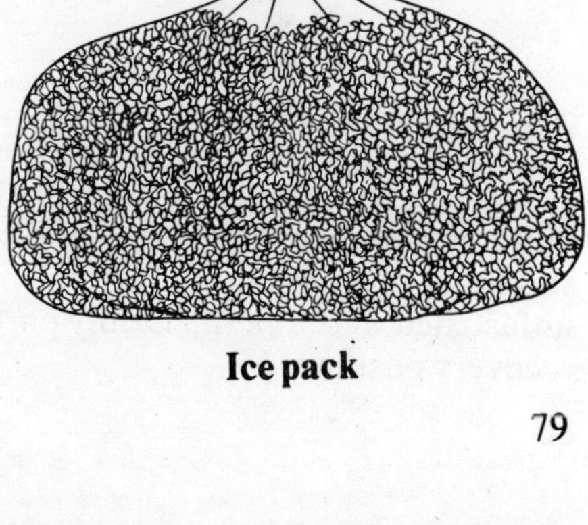

Ice pack

Cramp

When a muscle tightens and becomes hard it is painful. This pain is called muscle cramp, or simply, cramp. The way to get rid of a cramp is to break the tightness of the muscle by stretching it. Calf muscles that are cramped should be stretched by pulling the foot back and straightening the knee. The tightness and pain will quickly disappear. Fingers or toes that are cramped should be straightened and pulled back. Sometimes cramp is caused by a lack of salt, especially if the weather is hot and sticky. You sweat heavily and the body loses too much salt. In this case, put $\frac{1}{2}$ a teaspoonful of salt in a large tumbler of water and drink it.

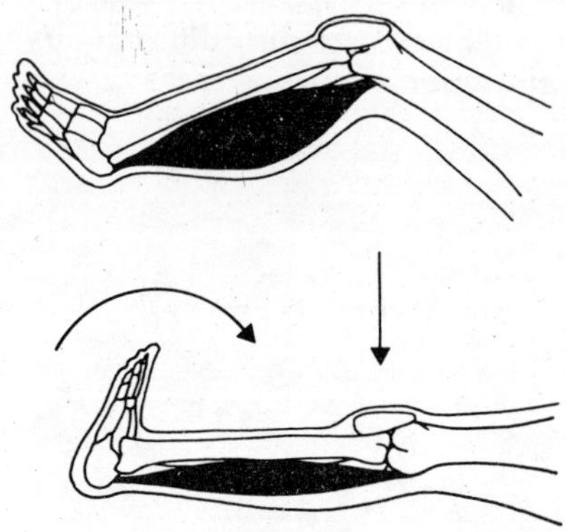

The cure for cramp is to stretch the muscle

Stitch

This is the name given to cramps of the belly and chest wall. They are usually caused by strenuous exercise such as running. The way to ease the pain is to stretch the muscles by rubbing the painful part.

Winding

A sharp blow in the 'stomach' may hit the major nerve centre in the abdomen—the solar plexus—and cause fainting and pain. The victim should be placed in a comfortable position and tight clothes unfastened. If the victim is only partially conscious, put him in the recovery position.

Hiccups

This is due to sudden contraction of the diaphragm which is a sheet of muscle separating the chest and abdomen. Thinking about it often makes it much worse. Distract the victim by having him sip water or take slow deep breaths. If the hiccups don't stop it may distress the person so much that a doctor will be needed.

Foreign bodies

When an object which does not belong to the body such as a safety pin, peanut or an insect gets into part of the body it is called a foreign body. It may produce pain, bleeding or irritation. In most cases it is best to remove the object, but if this cannot be done without causing further damage to the victim, leave it in position and call a doctor.

In the eye

Foreign body on the exposed part of the eye: Grit or insects often get into the eyes and cause irritation, redness and watering. Gently wipe the foreign body out with a wisp of cotton wool or the folded corner of a clean handkerchief.

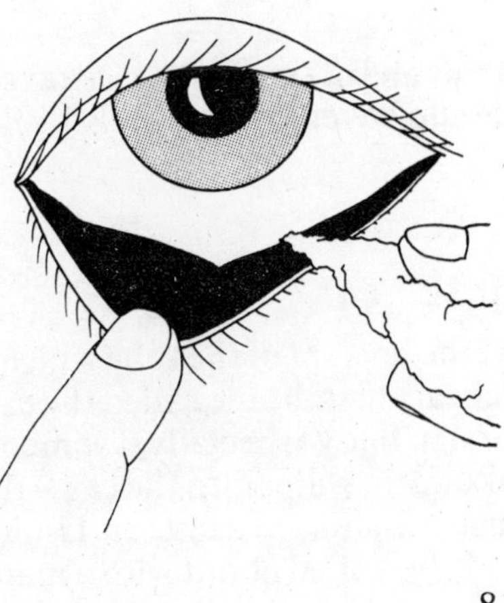

Foreign body under the lower eyelid: In this case pull the eyelid away and remove the foreign body in the same way described above.

Foreign body under the upper eyelid: The upper eyelid cannot be easily pulled away from the eye because it contains a tough inner layer of cartilage. It may be possible to remove the foreign body by placing the upper lid over the lower lid in such a way that the object comes off on the lower lid. If this fails, then place a hairgrip or matchstick along the top of the upper lid, flip the lid over and remove the foreign body.

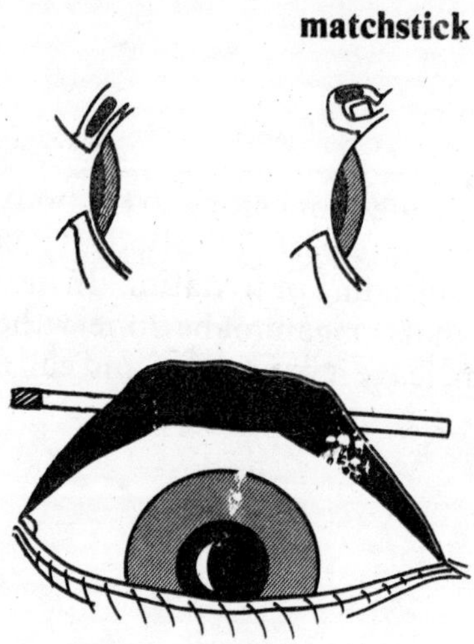

Acids and other caustic substances: If one of these gets into the eye it should be removed rapidly by flooding with water.

In the ear

At the bottom of the tube which leads from the outer ear there is a delicate membrane called the ear drum. This can be damaged by a foreign body especially if someone tries to poke the object out. Pour lukewarm water into the ear—this may remove the foreign body. If unsuccessful, see a doctor. Under no circumstance should the foreign body be poked about with a matchstick, tweezers, hairgrip, etc.

In the throat

Fishbones, peanuts and other pieces of food are the usual culprits in this case. The foreign body may irritate the throat and produce a tightening of the vocal cord muscles. This causes noisy and difficult breathing and the victim can easily suffocate. Help the victim to cough up the foreign body. This can be done by a sharp slap on the back between the shoulder blades. See Chapter 7.

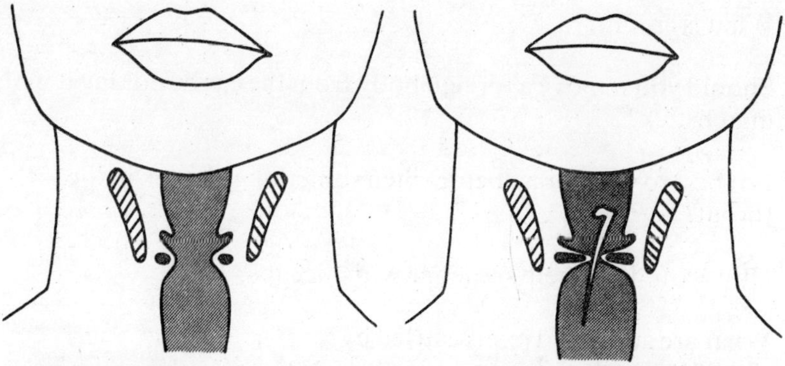

Throat clear
Vocal cord muscles relaxed
—breathing easy

Fishbone in throat
Vocal cord muscles tight
—breathing difficult

In the stomach

Occasionally a young child may swallow a nail or safety pin. This may puncture the wall of the stomach or guts. Get medical help immediately. Do not give anything by mouth as an operation may be needed to remove the unwanted object.

Quiz

1) What is a foreign body?

2) How would you relieve earache?

3) Describe the treatment for a black eye?

4) If bleach or another caustic substance gets into the eye, how would you deal with it?

5) What is cramp?

6) Should you remove a foreign body from the ear by poking it with a matchstick?

7) Is it best to wait for a doctor when something is stuck in the throat?

8) How would you help someone with hiccups?

9) What are aches and pains caused by?

10) Describe the way to stop cramp.

11 Dealing with disaster

A disaster in any situation in which one or more people are seriously injured. Disasters may occur in the home, at work, at school or on the road. When such injuries occur, the disaster may become much worse if no-one with any first aid skill or common sense is on the scene. There are many decisions to be made; expert help must be summoned, life-threatening injuries must be recognised and dealt with at once, people must be cared for and considered.

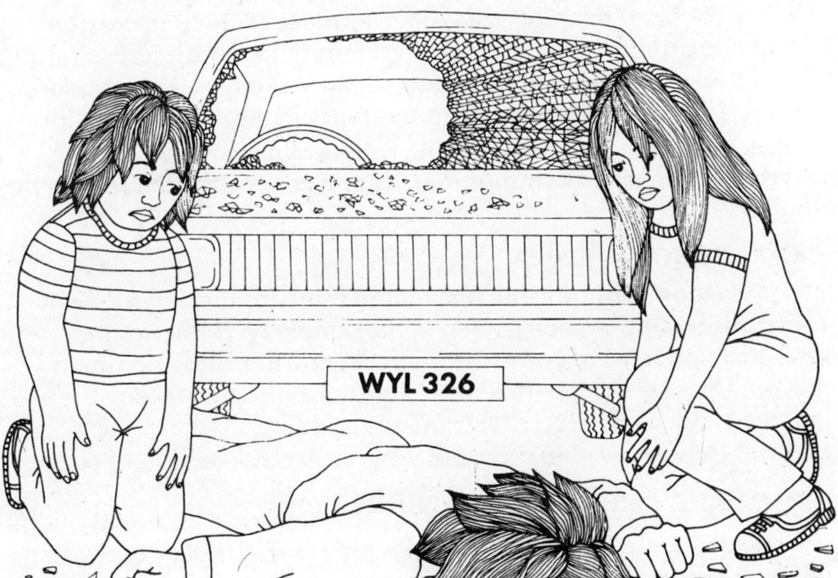

Calling for help

At any serious accident the injured will need expert medical help. The injuries or victims may be too many for you to handle alone.

TRY	to get onlookers to help
DIAL	999
ASK	for the ambulance service how long the ambulance will take to reach the accident time it will take to reach the hospital
GIVE	the telephone number from which you are calling address of the accident number of victims their injuries

What to do first

When there are several victims or several injuries and action is needed you must choose which job to do first. There are four conditions which need immediate treatment and they should be done in the following order:

1. When the heart has stopped—do external cardiac compression
2. When breathing has stopped—start mouth to mouth resuscitation
3. When an artery is bleeding—stop the flow of blood with pressure
4. When the casualty is unconscious—place in the recovery position

Quick action is the key to saving life. Because you cannot do everything at once, leave minor injuries and concentrate on life-saving jobs.

Searching for injuries

Unless you look methodically for signs of injury or disease, you will miss details. Examine each person in the same way. If the victim is conscious explain what you are doing, reassure him and ask him to help you. Do not forget to talk to the injured as they are often frightened and need to feel that someone is taking charge of the situation. Follow the plan opposite.

How people react and how to help

When involved in a serious accident people react in different ways. They get themselves into a "state".

State of fear: Fear or anxiety is probably the commonest reaction. It

Step One	See and recognise obvious injuries
Step Two	Check pulse breathing level of consciousness signs of bleeding
Step Three	Start at the head and work down to the toes. Take each limb in turn and then the chest and abdomen. } Look for bleeding, tenderness or signs of a fracture. If the victim is conscious talk to him as you do this
Step Four	Ask if the casualty is being seen by the doctor or treated for any disease. If the casualty is unconscious make a search for: Medic-alert Information Diabetic cards etc. The name and address of the victim.
Step Five	Always look for signs of shock
Step Six	Check and check again pulse breathing level of consciousness. Is bleeding controlled?

can be recognised by trembling, gooseflesh, a rapid heart beat and restlessness. It must be treated by calming the victim, talking gently and reassuringly. A warm blanket, a friendly face and as much good news as possible will provide much comfort.

State of grief: Another common reaction is sudden sadness or grief. In this situation the victim usually sobs or remains quiet and withdrawn. This responds to encouraging the victim to talk to you. Stay with him, listen to him, say as little as possible and do not pester him with needless questions.

State of excitement: When the victim gabbles uncontrollably and over-reacts to every stimulus he must be sheltered from the chaos and activity at the scene of the accident. Quiet, rest and firm instructions are necessary.

State of confusion: Any sudden event such as an accident especially after an injury to the head may make the casualty confused. This is easily recognised when the victim asks the same question time and time again, loses his grasp of the situation, or becomes disorientated. Such an injury needs a quiet situation and the constant reassuring presence of the same person.

State of forgetfulness: If the victim has forgotten how he became injured, what happened before or after the accident or even what his name and address is, you should make a special note of this. It probably indicates concussion and he should certainly see a doctor.

At a road accident

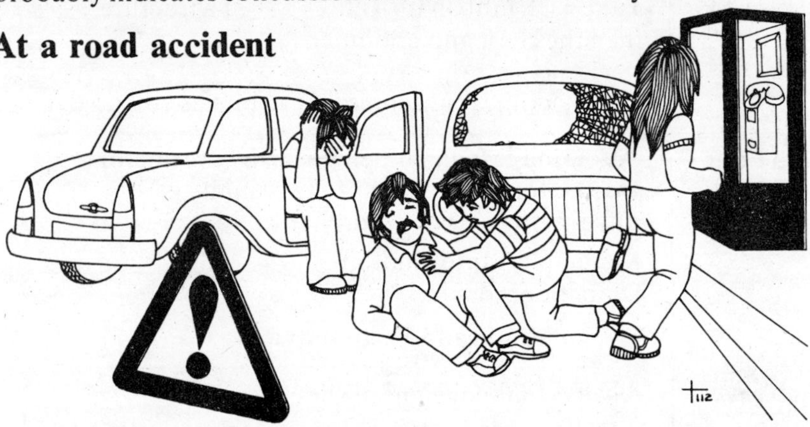

Redirect traffic: Do not rush on to the road without first making sure that it is safe to cross. Switch off the car's engine and disconnect the battery if possible. Set reflective triangles or other warning devices some 50 metres on both sides of the accident. If there is fast moving traffic on the road the warning triangles should be moved even further from the crash.

Send for help

Check the victim: If he is not breathing start immediate mouth to mouth resuscitation: if the heart has stopped initiate external cardiac compression.

Do not move the victim: Unless the car is on fire, he is in danger of being hit by oncoming traffic, or his breathing or heart has stopped, the victim should not be disturbed.

Do not smoke: Petrol may have spilled on the roadway and the cigarette could cause a fire or explosion.

Do not give alcohol: This would not help the victim medically and the police might think he had been drinking while driving.

Fire

A fire extinguisher, blanket or earth may be used to fight a fire, but an explosion may occur. If there is a fire move yourself and the victim away immediately. Never use water as this may spread the flames.

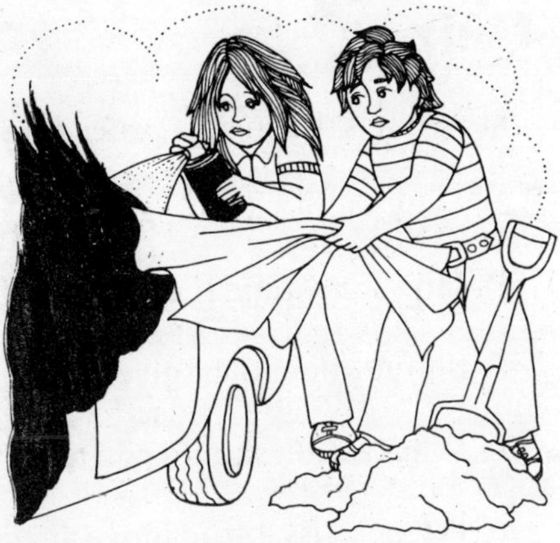

Trapped victim

Check his respiration and pulse. If he is not breathing, start immediate mouth to mouth resuscitation. If the heart has stopped do not waste a lot of time trying to free him from the wreck but begin external cardiac compression. Delay will most certainly result in the victim's death. It may be difficult to perform the external cardiac compression properly, but do the best you can.

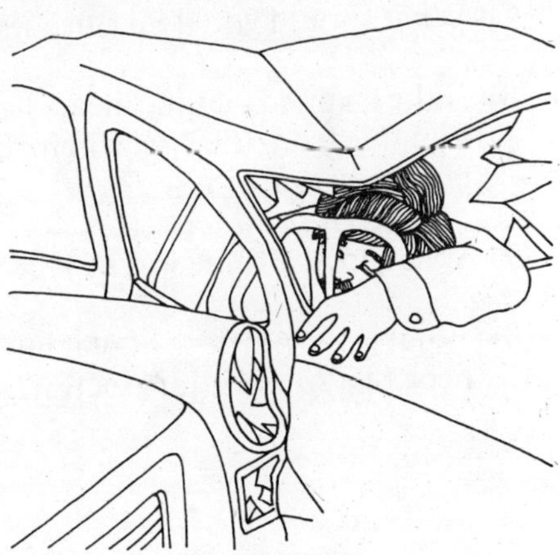

Spinal injury

Is the victim complaining of a pain in the back?
Does he have difficulty in moving his fingers or toes?
Has any part of his body become numb?
If so, it is likely that there has been an injury to the spine. A common site of such injuries at a road accident is in the neck. Roll up a newspaper and secure it round the neck with string to reduce the possibility of further injury. Do not move the victim unless it is absolutely necessary to do so, as this could cause further injury which could lead to paralysis.

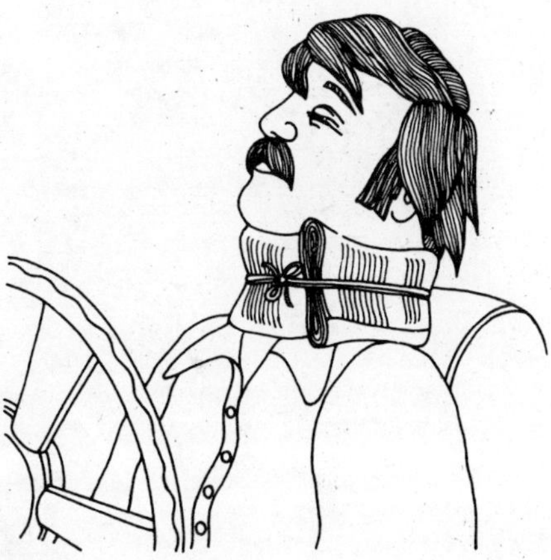

Quiz

1) What is the correct procedure at a road accident?

2) Why should warning devices be placed on the road?

3) How far should they be from the crash site?

4) Should alcohol be given to the victim?

5) What action should you take if breathing has stopped?

6) Is it permissable to move an unconscious victim?

7) What should you do if a fire starts in one of the cars?

8) If the trapped victim's heart has stopped beating, should you pull him free from the wreck before beginning external cardiac compression?

9) What are the three ways to recognise injuries to the spine?

10) What is the purpose of placing a rolled up newspaper around the neck of a spinal injury victim?

The Appendices

Appendix 1

Applying a bandage

Bandages are strips of material used to bind up injuries. They are usually made from gauze, linen, crepe or elastic, but in an emergency any material will do; a sheet, pillow case or shirt torn into strips, for example, will bind the wound just as effectively as bandages bought from a Chemist.

Bandages are used for: keeping dressings in place
applying pressure to bleeding or swollen parts
holding a limb or part of the body still
giving support to injured joints.

Dressings are materials which are put directly onto a wound. They should always be very clean and, if possible, sterile to prevent infection. If a proper sterile gauze dressing is not available then the inside of a clean handkerchief will do.

Dressings are used to: stop bleeding
prevent germs entering the wound
soaking up body fluids or infected materi[al]
from the wound.

Bandaging is a skill which can only be mastered by practice and by watching other people. Here are a few tips to help you:

Always use a suitably sized bandage e.g. a small (one inch) bandage for a finger or a large (six inch) bandage for a thigh.

Roll from the inside to the outside, holding the head of the bandage

Start at the narrowest part and work towards the widest part.

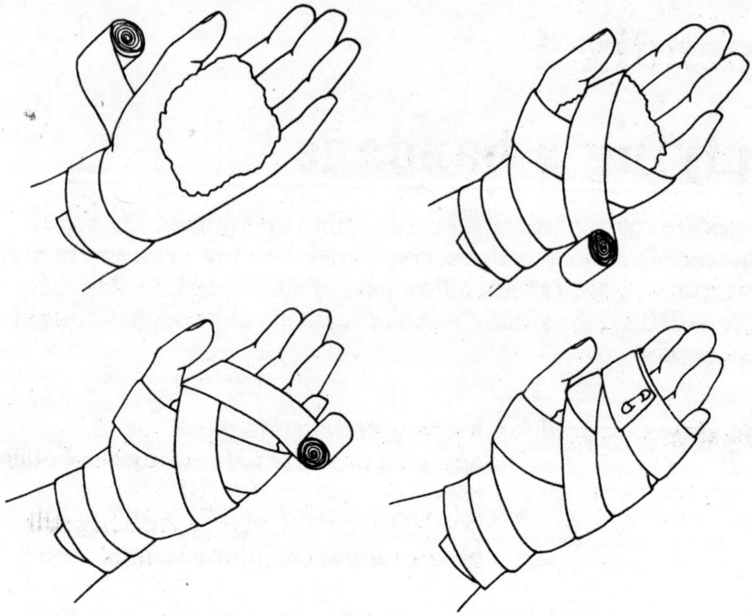

A two-inch bandage for the hand

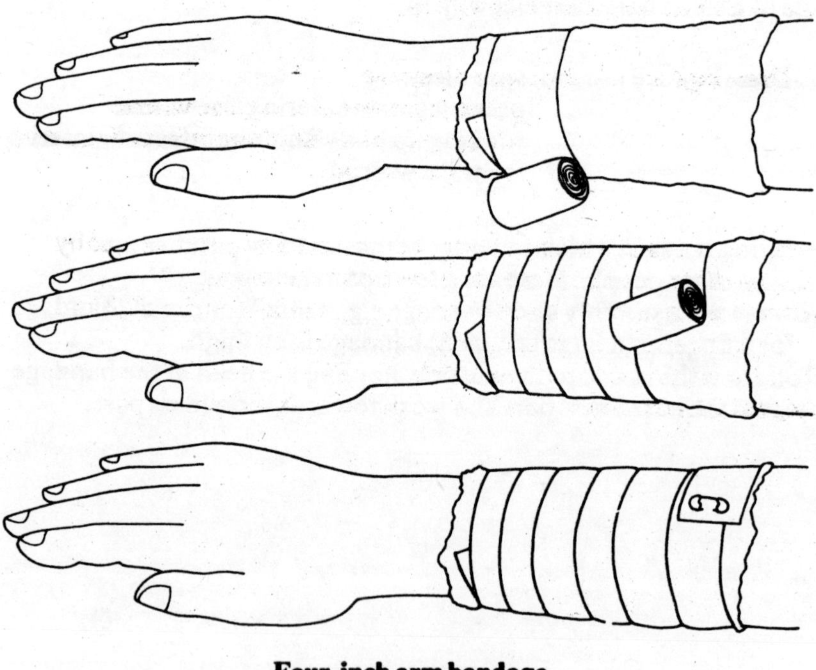

Four-inch arm bandage

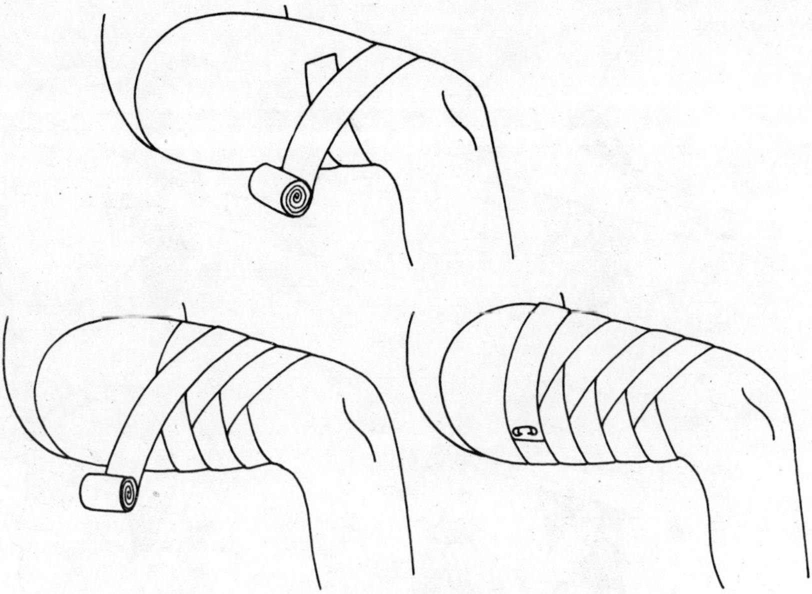

A six-inch roller bandage for the thigh

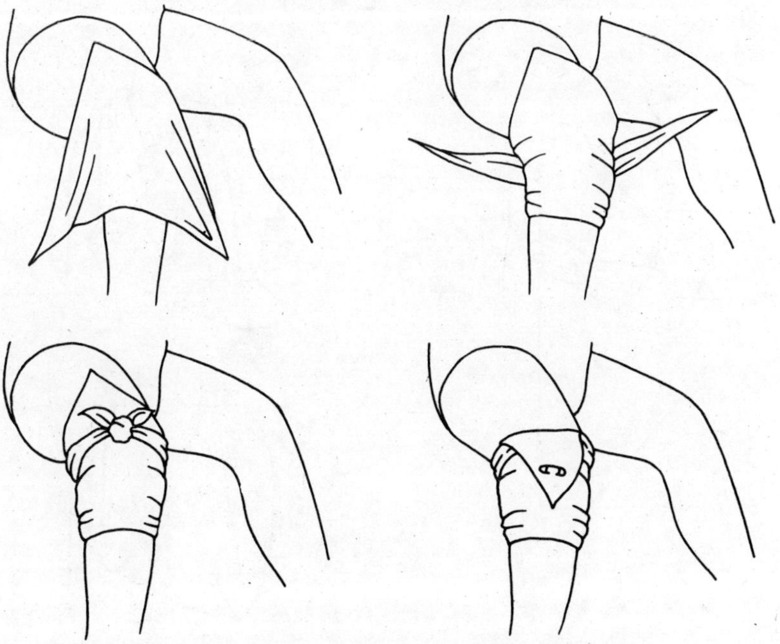

Triangular bandage around the knee

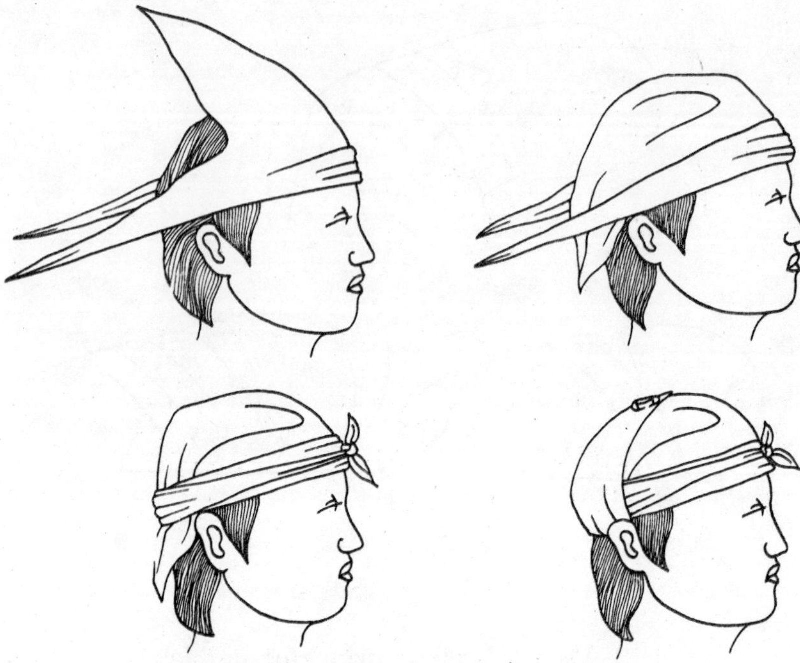

Binding the head with a triangular bandage

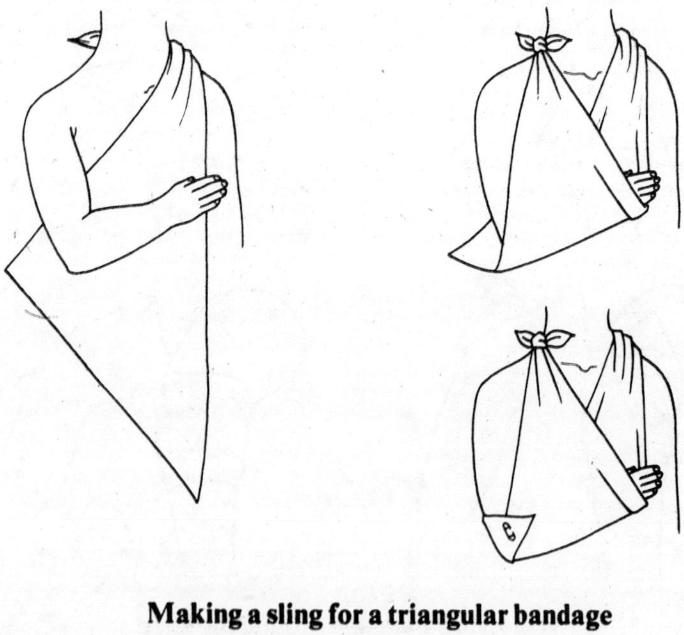

Making a sling for a triangular bandage

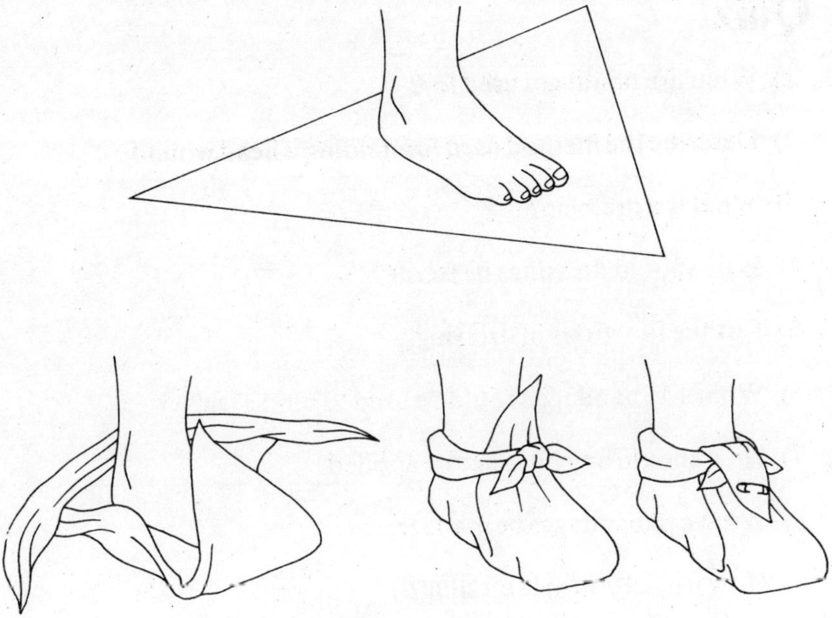

Bandaging the foot

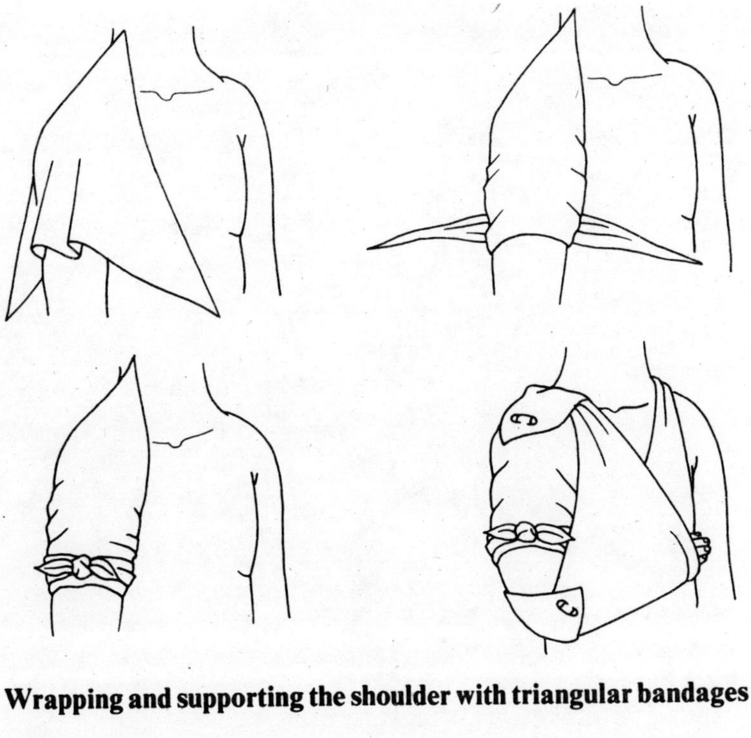

Wrapping and supporting the shoulder with triangular bandages

Quiz

1) What are bandages used for?

2) Describe the method used for binding a head wound.

3) What is a dressing?

4) Why should dressings be sterile?

5) List the functions of dressings.

6) What size bandage should be used to bind a leg?

7) How should any bandage be applied?

8) What can bandages be made from?

9) How would you make a sling?

10) Describe the method for bandaging a hand wound.

Appendix 2

Dealing with a fracture

When a bone is broken the ends cut into the flesh producing pain and further injury. It is therefore important to stop the bone from altering its position and this is best done by preventing movement at the joints above and below the break. A variety of materials can be used for the job; slings, splints, padding and bandages, for example:

Slings: usually made from a triangular bandage, slings can be used to support broken or badly bruised arms.

Splints: used to keep arms or legs immobilised, splints are made from rigid lengths of wood or metal.

Padding: wads of soft material, this is used to stop bony points or injured parts rubbing together.

Bandages: these are strips of material, used to tie splints and padding in place.

Details of how to deal with individual fractures follows in the next few pages. Here are a few points to remember as you go through them:

Never tie a knot over an injured part.

Always place padding around the injury and between bony parts.

Use splints if they are available. If they are not, the injured part may be immobilised by binding it to another part of the body.

Do not get carried away dealing with broken bones and forget the rest of the victim's injuries.

Always handle a broken limb gently.

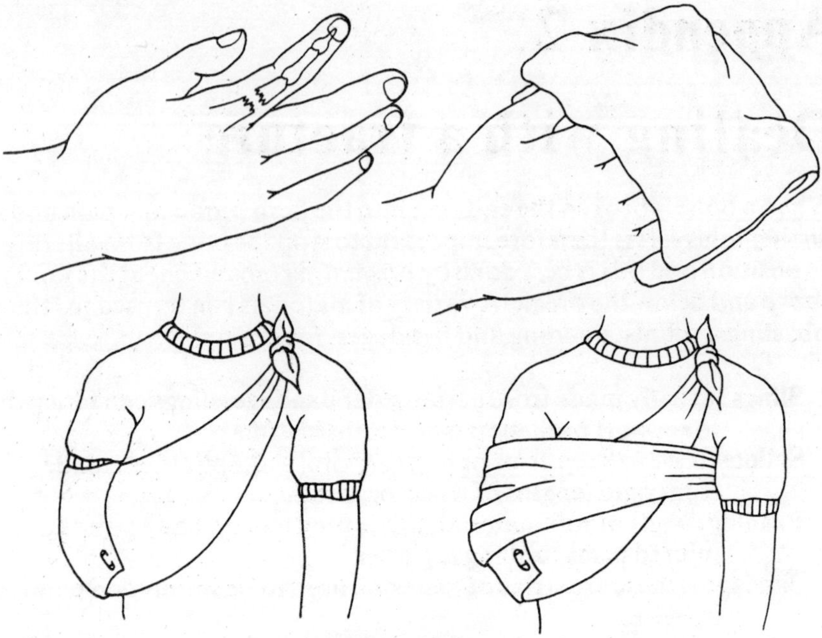

A bróken finger

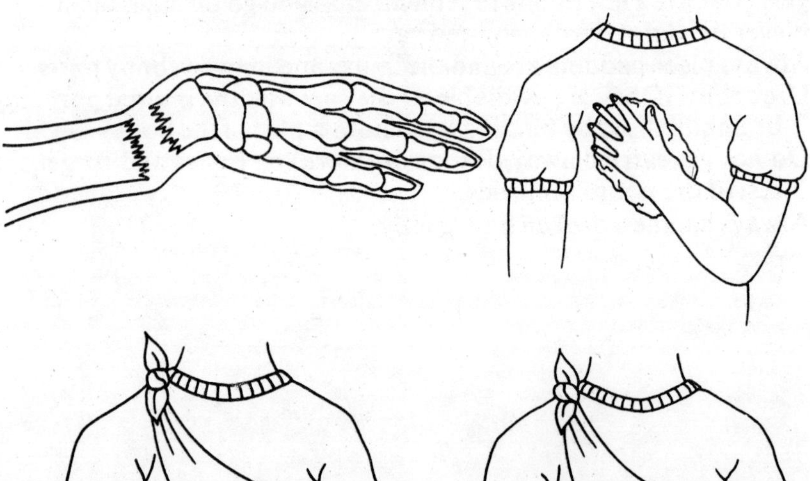

Fractured wrist

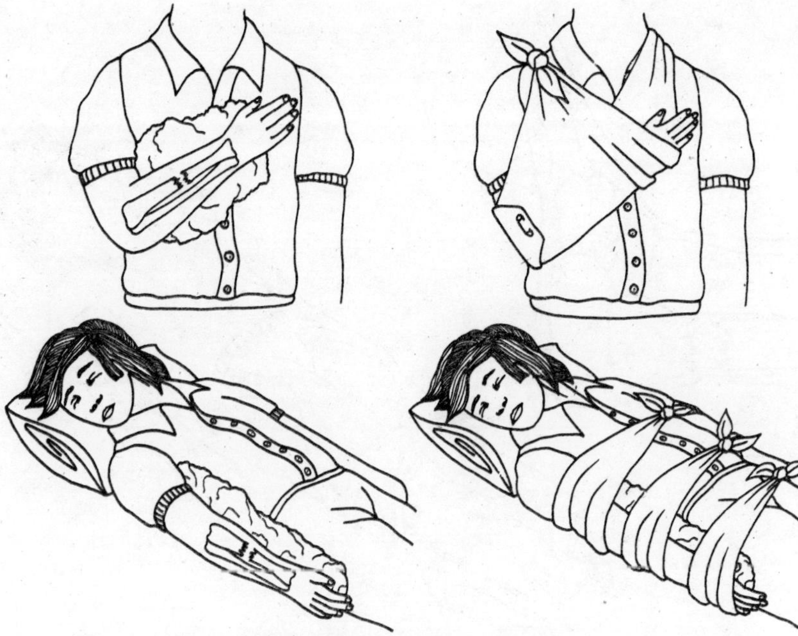

A break in the bone of the arm

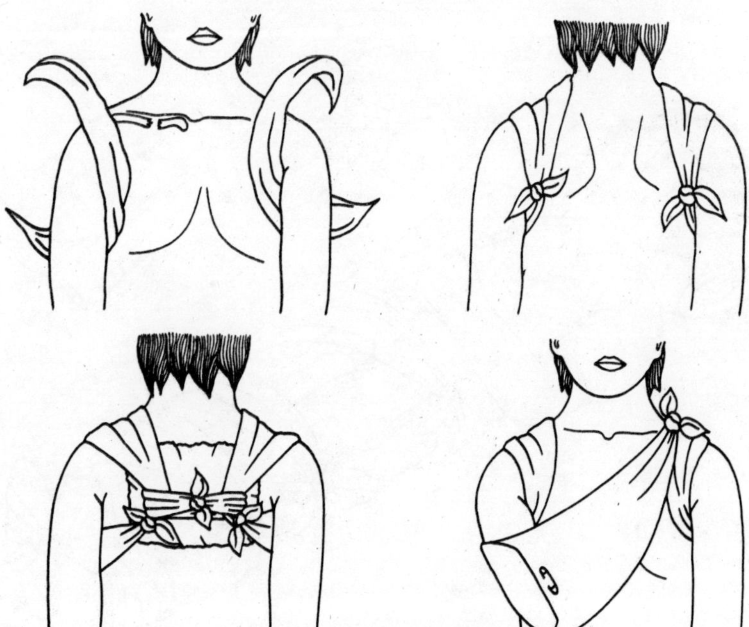

Cracked collar bone

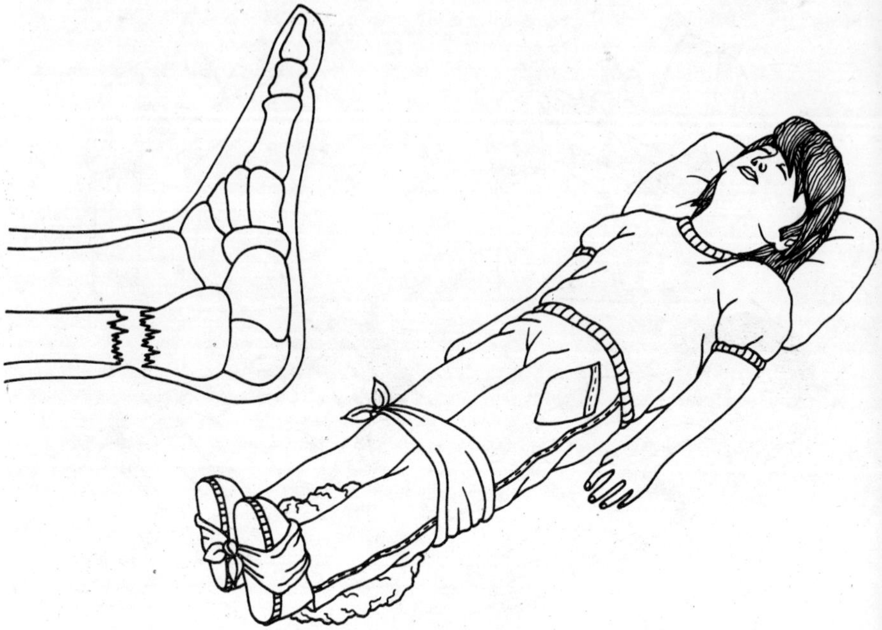

A fractured ankle

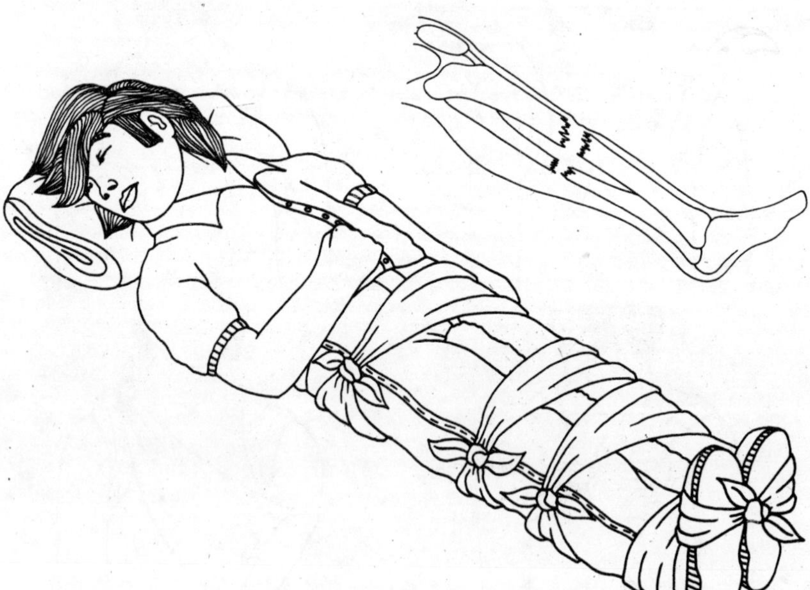

Broken leg

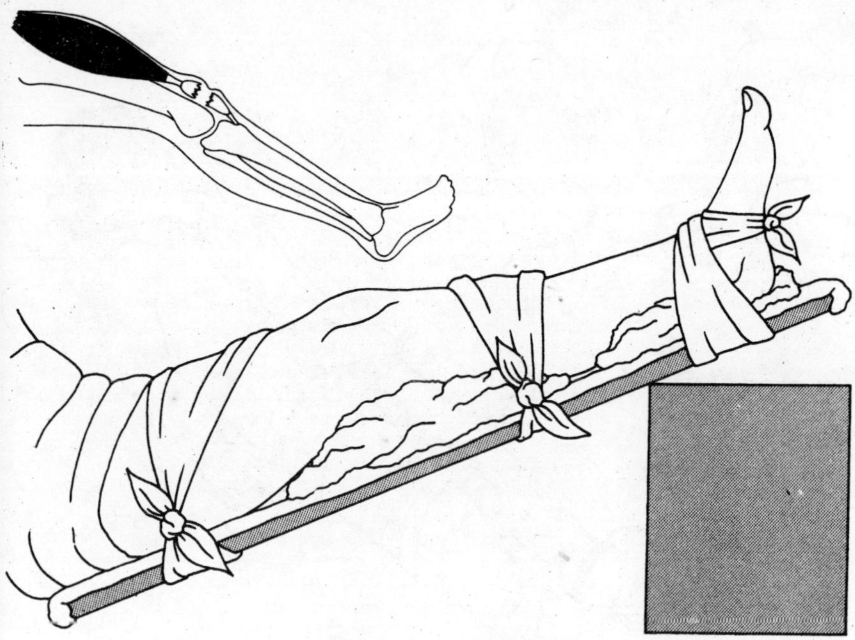

A broken knee cap

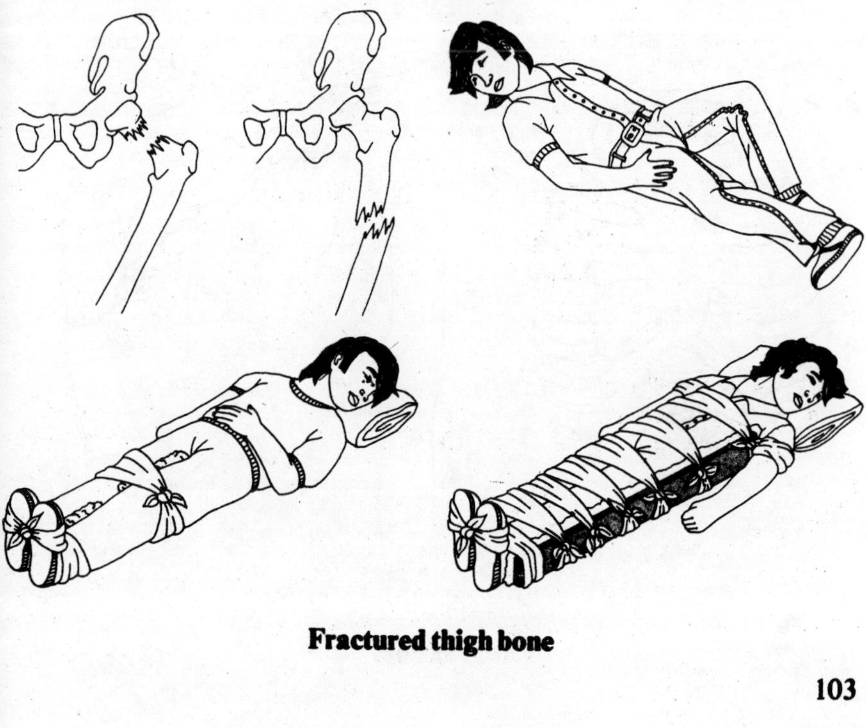

Fractured thigh bone

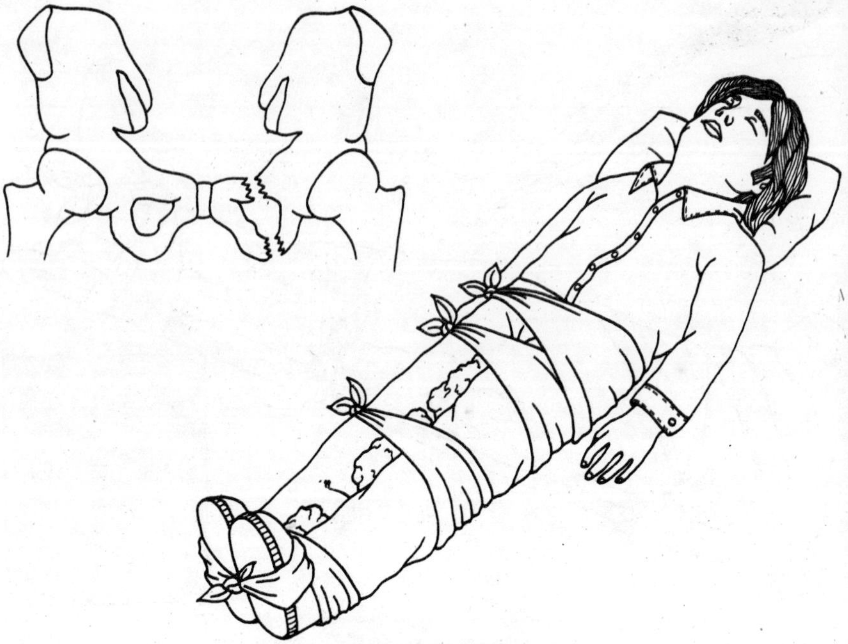

Fractured hip bone

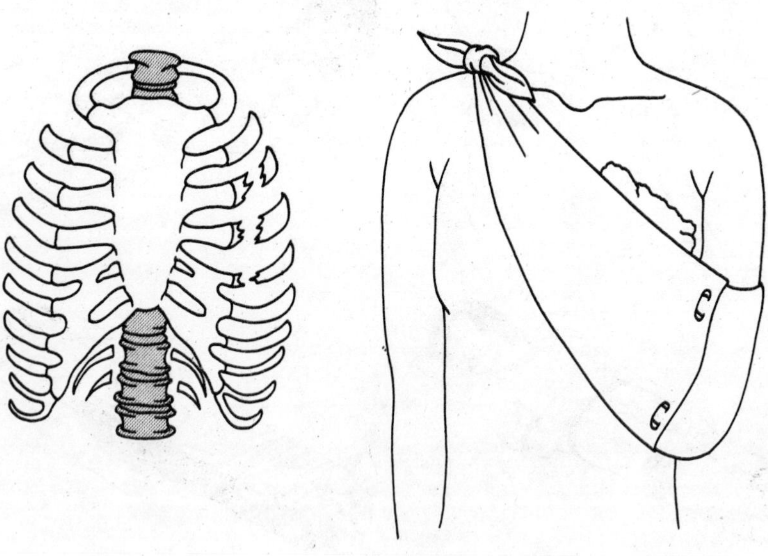

Cracked ribs

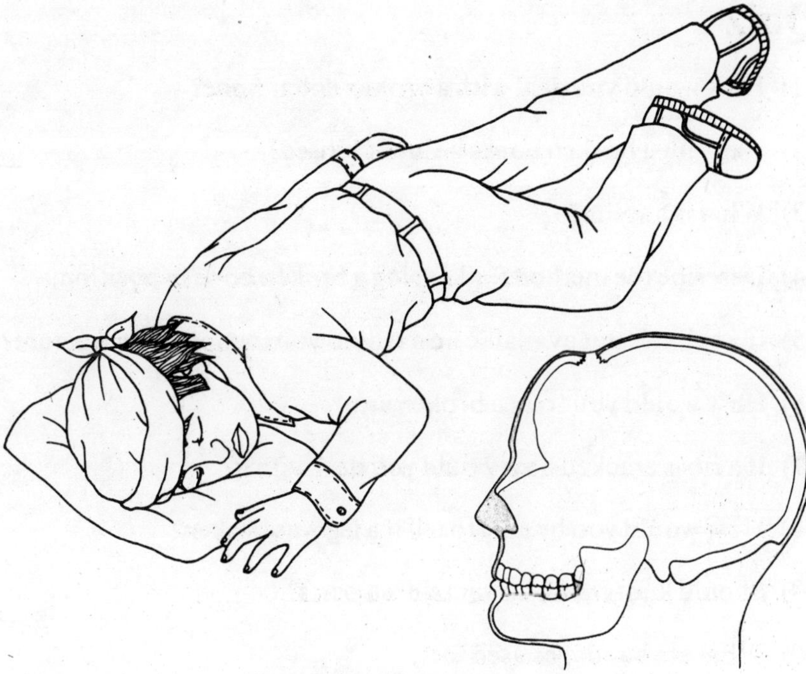

A fractured skull

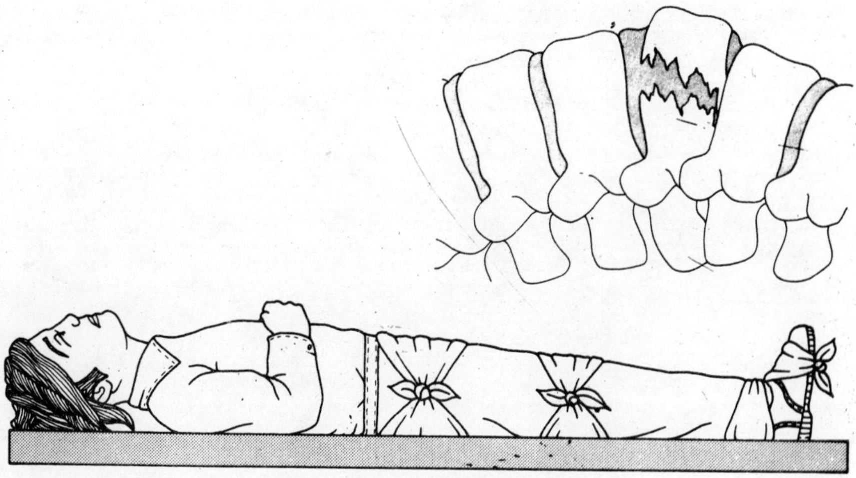

Broken spine

Quiz

1) How would you deal with a broken collar bone?

2) Why must broken bones be immobilised?

3) What is a splint?

4) Describe the method for keeping a broken bone in position.

5) If a splint is not available how would you immobilise a fracture?

6) How would you treat a broken arm?

7) If a rib is cracked how would you deal with it?

8) How would you be able to tell if a leg was broken?

9) Should knots be tied over injured parts?

10) What are bandages used for?

Appendix 3

Carrying the victim

First aid is only the first step in treating an injured person. The victim must often be taken from the scene of the accident to a hospital or doctor and this must be done in such a way that no further injury occurs while the person is being moved. This is difficult and there is a correct way in which to help the victim in each case, depending on the type of injury. The methods are designed to reduce pain and suffering:

Remember: to keep injured parts still
to keep the injured person warm
to keep the victim in a comfortable position.

The victim's condition may improve or deteriorate during the time spent transporting him to a doctor. It is therefore important to take regular checks of his pulse, breathing and state of consciousness, and note these down on a piece of paper, as they may be useful later.
If you are dealing with a serious condition do not be afraid of calling an ambulance. Dial 999 from the nearest telephone. You do not need any money to do this. When the telephone operator answers tell her which emergency service you need: fire, police or ambulance, and exactly where the accident has occurred (see chapter 11).

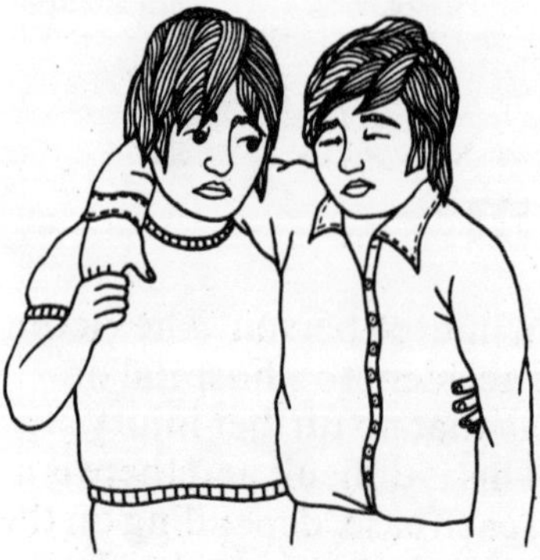

Human crutch

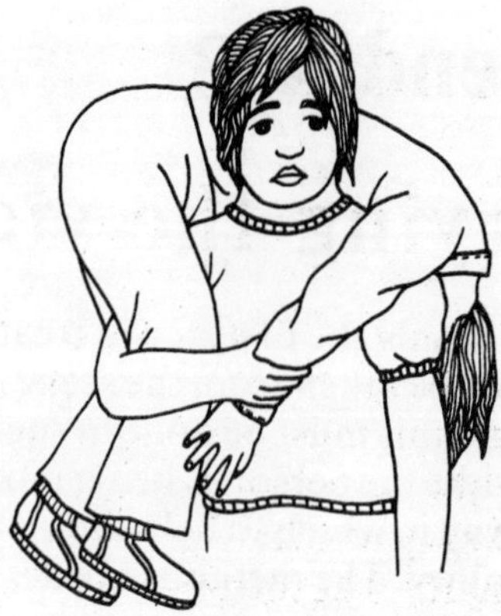

Fireman's lift

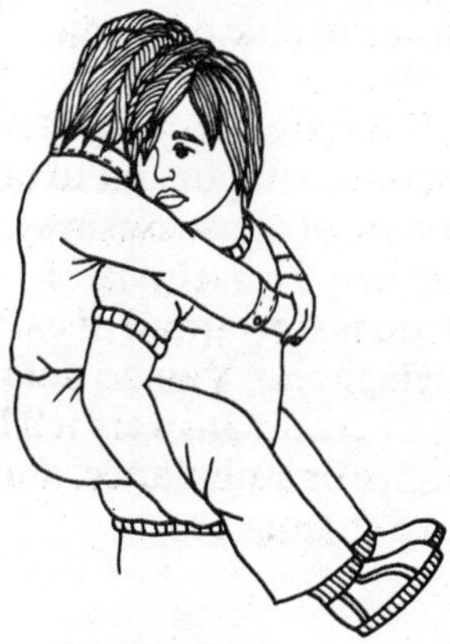

Pick-a-back

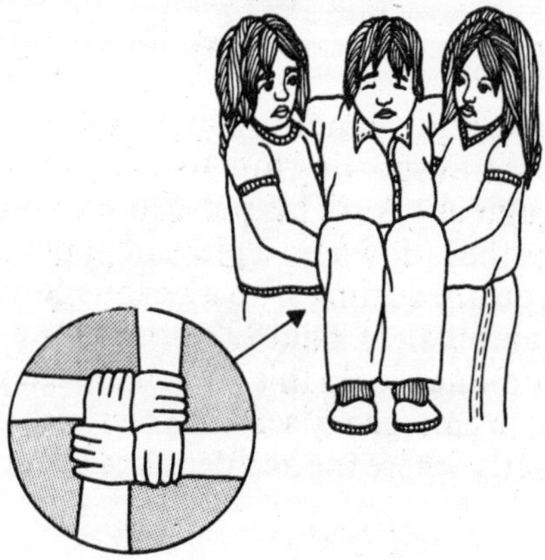

Four-handed seat

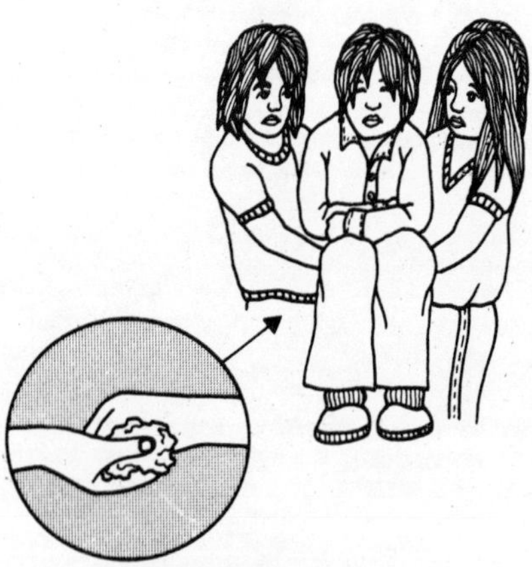

Two-handed seat

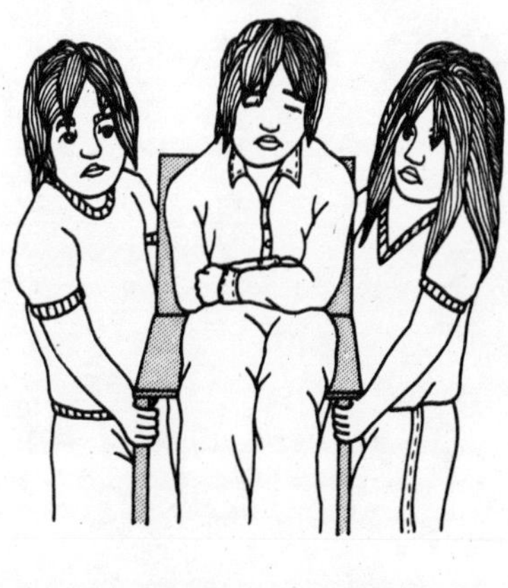

Kitchen-chair lift

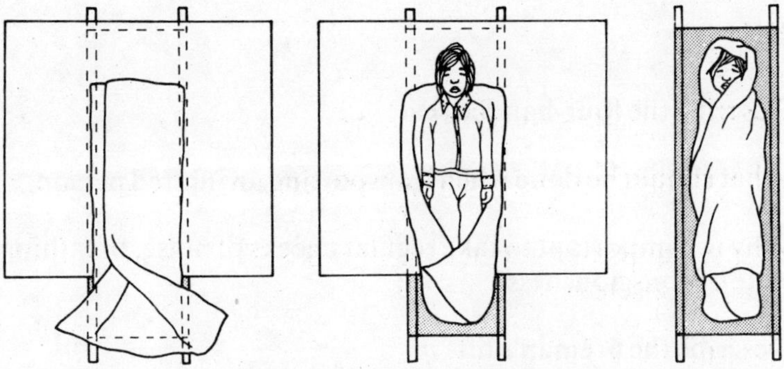

The two-blanket stretcher

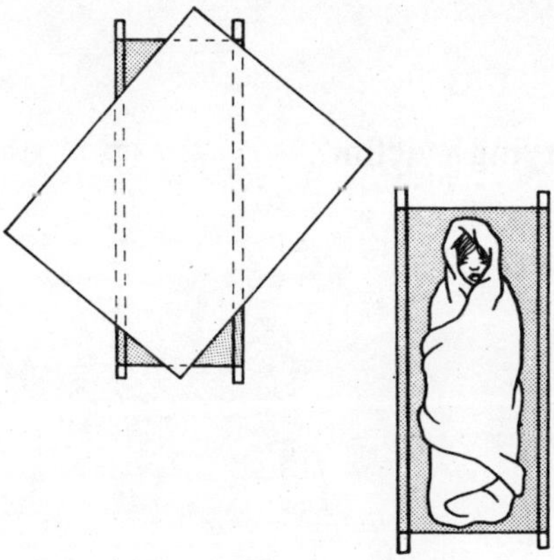

One-blanket stretcher

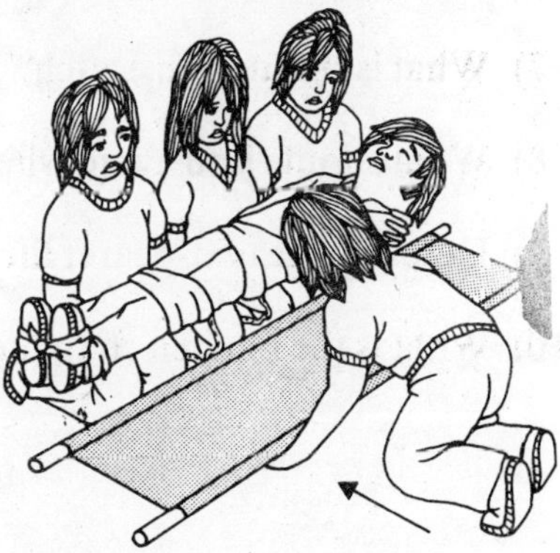

Four people load a stretcher

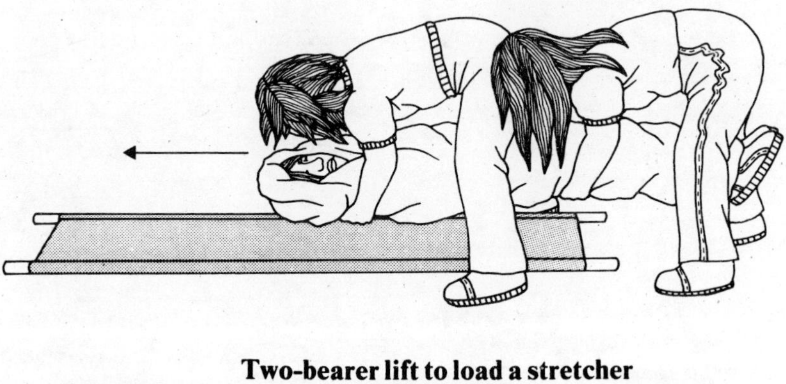

Two-bearer lift to load a stretcher

Quiz

1) Describe the four-handed seat.

2) What should be done when transporting an injured person.

3) Why is it important to take regular checks of pulse, breathing and state of consciousness?

4) Describe the fireman's lift.

5) How can a victim be lifted on to a stretcher?

6) How can you get help in an emergency?

7) What is the human crutch?

8) What should you avoid when carrying a victim?

9) Describe the two-bearer lift.

10) What is the kitchen chair method?

Appendix 4

Using the right word: a guide to first aid terms

Airway: name given to the passages which connect the lungs to the atmosphere outside the body.

Angina: pain produced by the heart; a severe crushing pain in the centre of the chest or strangling sensation in the throat.

Apoplexy: old fashioned name for a stroke or bleeding in the brain.

Artery: blood vessel which takes blood from the heart to the rest of the body.

Artificial Respiration: method of helping the victim to breath; this is best done by the mouth to mouth method.

Asphyxia: out of date term for breathing with difficulty, which leads to shortage of oxygen, an excess of carbon dioxide in the blood and eventual suffocation.

Asthma: condition which makes breathing difficult, often accompanied by a wheeze.

Bandage: strip of cloth or other material used to bind up a wound.

Blood: red fluid which circulates in the arteries and veins of the body transporting oxygen and food stuffs and removing waste materials.

Brachial Artery: the main blood vessel of the arm.

Capillary: minute blood vessels between the ends of the arteries and the beginnings of the veins.

Carbon Dioxide: waste gas produced by the body and exhaled through the lungs and air passages.

Carbon Monoxide: poisonous gas produced by car and other internal combustion engines and in some domestic gas supplies. It is extremely dangerous and, if inhaled, can kill.

Carotid Artery: main artery in the neck.

Circulation: system through which blood moves around the body.

Coma: unconscious state from which it is impossible to rouse a person.

Convulsion: fit or sudden loss of consciousness often associated with shaking of whole or part of the body.

Cyanosis: blueness of the lips or finger tips produced by shortage of oxygen in the blood, or poor blood circulation.

Diabetes: disease in which the body's ability to use sugar is impaired due to insufficient insulin. This results in a high concentration of sugar in the blood and urine.

Diagnosis: process of deciding on the nature and name of the condition or disease from which a person is suffering.

Digestion: breaking up of food substances in the gut before absorption into the body.

Dislocation: bones that are out of joint.

Dressing: sterile or very clean piece of material for application directly onto a wound.

Drug: another word for a medicine or substance intended for healing; not all drugs are addictive.

Emetic: substance to make a casualty vomit (such as salt and water or Ipecac syrup).

Epilepsy: disease in which the sufferer suddenly loses consciousness or has a fit.

Exposure: condition produced when the body's temperature regulation mechanism fails and the person becomes too hot or too cold.

Faint: weak, dizzy feeling followed by a short loss of consciousness due to poor blood supply to the brain.

Femoral Artery: the main blood vessel in the leg.

Fit: loss of consciousness due to an electrical discharge in the brain.

Fracture: break or crack in a bone.

Haemoglobin: red pigment in the blood cells which combines readily with oxygen.

Heart Attack: sudden crushing pain in the chest, due to inadequate blood supply to the heart muscle.

Hypothermia: loss of body heat producing a severe fall in body temperature.

Hysteria: an uncontrolled emotion occurring in immature people.

Insulin: chemical substance in the body which regulates the concentration of sugar in the blood.

Joint: structure at which bones are joined together.

Kidneys: pair of organs in the body which filter chemicals, retaining some and passing others out in the urine.

Larynx: the voice box or Adam's Apple.

Ligament: tough tissue which binds together bodily structures such as bones.

Lungs: two air-filled, sac-like organs in the chest through which oxygen is inhaled and carbon dioxide exhaled.

Medic-Alert: disc or bracelet worn by people with certain illnesses such as epilepsy or diabetes, which gives vital information about the person.

Muscles: bundles of special fibres which change length producing movement.

Nerves: collections of fibres which carry "electrical" impulses around the body.

Oesophagus: tube of muscular tissue connecting the mouth to the stomach.

Oxygen: gas, vital to the body's production of energy, making up one-fifth of the air.

Pharynx: space at the back of the nose and mouth.

Poison: any substance which is harmful to the body.

Pulse: throbbing of the arteries due to the pumping of blood by the heart.

Radial Artery: main artery on the thumb side of the wrist.

Resuscitation: attempt to restart a stopped heart or restore breathing.

Shock: reaction of the body in which all the tissues are starved of oxygen.

Sign: cluc noticed by a doctor or first-aider which indicates the cause of illness (c.f. symptoms).

Sling: material used to hold an injured limb.

Sprain: stretched ligament.

Strain: stretched muscle or tendon.

Stroke: illness produced by the loss of blood supply to an area of the brain.

Sterile: germ-free condition.

Stupor: a level of unconsciousness in which only pain produces a reaction.

Symptom: clue noticed by the sufferer which indicates the cause of illness. (c.f. sign)

Temperature: degree of heat in the body. The normal temperature of the body is 37°C or 98·4°F.

Thorax: the space surrounded by the ribs, separated from the abdomen by the diaphragm and containing the heart, lungs and oesophagus.

Tissue: structures from which the body is made such as muscle, bone and fat.

Urine: liquid waste material produced by the kidneys.

Vein: thin-walled tube carrying blood towards the heart.

Wound: hole in the skin produced by an injury.

The final test
Multiple choice quiz

Now you have come to the end of the book test yourself with the following twenty questions. The questions are followed by five statements which are either true or false. In each case, tick the correct box and if you do not know the answer leave it blank. When you have finished, turn to the next page for the correct answers. For each correct answer give yourself one mark.

Ratings: 100–75 Excellent
75–50 Good
50–25 Poor
25–0 Very poor.

1. What is the purpose of first aid? *Yes* *No*

A. To preserve life ☐ ☐
B. To learn biology ☐ ☐
C. To learn bandaging ☐ ☐
D. To prevent further injury ☐ ☐
E. To promote recovery ☐ ☐

2. Which of the following can be given a drink?

A. Someone with a broken thigh bone ☐ ☐
B. A person who is poisoned with acid ☐ ☐
C. Someone who is in shock ☐ ☐
D. Someone with very severe stomach pains ☐ ☐
E. Someone poisoned with aspirin ☐ ☐

3. What is the correct treatment of a burn?

A. Applying a soothing ointment ☐ ☐
B. Making the victim vomit ☐ ☐
C. Covering the burn with a sterile dressing ☐ ☐
D. Running the burned part under cold water for one minute ☐ ☐
E. Running the burned part under cold water for ten minutes ☐ ☐

4. Which of the following statements are true?

A. A sprain is a stretched ligament ☐ ☐
B. A strain is a stretched ligament ☐ ☐
C. The hip joint rarely dislocates ☐ ☐
D. The shoulder joint may dislocate ☐ ☐
E. A sprained ankle joint should be treated by exercise ☐ ☐

5. Which of the following are true of a fracture?

A. They never occur in short bones ☐ ☐
B. The broken ends of bones may cause pain ☐ ☐
C. Swelling is rare ☐ ☐
D. There may be some unusual movement ☐ ☐
E. A fracture should be treated by immobilisation ☐ ☐

6. Which of the following may produce coma? *Yes* *No*

A. Head injury ☐ ☐
B. Diabetes ☐ ☐
C. Epilepsy ☐ ☐
D. A stroke ☐ ☐
E. Sunstroke ☐ ☐

7. Which of the following are signs of brain compression?

A. Flushed complexion ☐ ☐
B. Rapid pulse ☐ ☐
C. Unequal pupil sizes ☐ ☐
D. Pale complexion ☐ ☐
E. Numbness down one side of the body ☐ ☐

8. Which of the following suggest an insulin reaction (hypoglycaemic attack)?

A. Sweating and trembling ☐ ☐
B. Rapid loss of consciousness ☐ ☐
C. A fruity smell on the breath ☐ ☐
D. A drunken appearance ☐ ☐
E. Slow pulse ☐ ☐

9. How would you treat cold exhaustion?

A. Give a drink of brandy ☐ ☐
B. Protect the victim from the wind ☐ ☐
C. Keep the victim dry ☐ ☐
D. Reheat rapidly ☐ ☐
E. Warm gradually ☐ ☐

10. In the case of a drowned casualty should you:

A. Turn the victim upside down to drain water from the lungs? ☐ ☐
B. Bend the head forward and blow air into the lungs? ☐ ☐
C. Clear the mouth, pull the head back and blow into the lungs? ☐ ☐
D. Not attempt to give artificial respiration because the lungs are full of water? ☐ ☐
E. Not take the pulse because you are wasting time? ☐ ☐

11. When you are resuscitating a victim you should: *Yes No*

A. Perform external cardiac compression 15 times a minute ☐ ☐
B. Perform external cardiac compression 60 times a minute ☐ ☐
C. Perform mouth to mouth resuscitation 15 times a minute ☐ ☐
D. Perform mouth to mouth resuscitation 60 times a minute ☐ ☐
E. Continue until you are exhausted. ☐ ☐

12. Which of the following statements are true?

A. The body contains five litres of blood ☐ ☐
B. The pulse slows when blood is lost ☐ ☐
C. Shock may result from blood loss ☐ ☐
D. Bleeding is always confined to the outside of the body ☐ ☐
E. A fractured bone may cause bleeding ☐ ☐

13. How should you stop bleeding?

A. Apply a tourniquet ☐ ☐
B. Apply direct pressure to the bleeding point ☐ ☐
C. Elevate the limb and lie the victim down ☐ ☐
D. Lower the limbs and sit the victim upright ☐ ☐
E. If the bleeding does not stop apply pressure to an artery ☐ ☐

14. The following may stop the heart beating

A. Sunburn ☐ ☐
B. Electric shock ☐ ☐
C. Heart attack ☐ ☐
D. Stroke ☐ ☐
E. Hysterical fit ☐ ☐

15. External cardiac compression:

A. Squeezes the heart between the breastbone and backbone ☐ ☐
B. Must always be done gently ☐ ☐
C. Should be preceded by a sharp blow on the chest ☐ ☐
D. Must be performed with the casualty on a hard surface ☐ ☐
E. Must not break ribs ☐ ☐

16. Foreign bodies: *Yes* *No*

A. Must always be removed from a wound ☐ ☐
B. Those in the ear canal should not be removed ☐ ☐
C. In the throat may be removed by drinking olive oil ☐ ☐
D. In the eye should be removed by a salt solution ☐ ☐
E. Such as an open safety pin swallowed into the stomach should be removed by making the victim sick ☐ ☐

17. In the case of suspected spinal injury at a road traffic accident:

A. The victim should be lifted gently from the wreck and placed on the road ☐ ☐
B. Should not be given alcohol ☐ ☐
C. Injury to the spine may be indicated by unequal size of the pupils ☐ ☐
D. The victim should not be moved at any cost ☐ ☐
E. External cardiac compression should not be carried out ☐ ☐

18. Which of the following definitions is true?

A. "Drugs" are addictive and poisonous substances banned by law ☐ ☐
B. "Medic-alert" is a name for a medical emergency ☐ ☐
C. "Airways" is a name given to special radio waves ☐ ☐
D. "Exposure" is the result of the breakdown of the body's heat regulation mechanism ☐ ☐
E. "Dislocation" is another way of saying "out of joint" ☐ ☐

19. Bandages have the following uses:

A. To keep a dressing in place ☐ ☐
B. To apply pressure to a bleeding wound ☐ ☐
C. To cut off blood supply to a limb ☐ ☐
D. To support an injured limb ☐ ☐
E. To immobilise a broken limb ☐ ☐

20. The following are true of shock:

A. May be due to loss of blood ☐ ☐
B. Is shown by a fast fading pulse ☐ ☐
C. Should be treated by a drink of hot tea ☐ ☐
D. The face is usually flushed ☐ ☐
E. The victim should be laid flat to improve the blood circulation ☐ ☐

The final test

		Yes	No
1.	a)	☒	☐
	b)	☐	☒
	c)	☐	☒
	d)	☒	☐
	e)	☒	☐
2.	a)	☐	☒
	b)	☒	☐
	c)	☐	☒
	d)	☐	☒
	e)	☒	☐
3.	a)	☐	☒
	b)	☐	☒
	c)	☒	☐
	d)	☐	☒
	e)	☒	☐
4.	a)	☒	☐
	b)	☐	☒
	c)	☒	☐
	d)	☒	☐
	e)	☐	☒
5.	a)	☐	☒
	b)	☒	☐
	c)	☐	☒
	d)	☒	☐
	e)	☒	☐
6.	a)	☒	☐
	b)	☒	☐
	c)	☒	☐
	d)	☒	☐
	e)	☒	☐
7.	a)	☒	☐
	b)	☐	☒
	c)	☒	☐
	d)	☐	☒
	e)	☒	☐
8.	a)	☒	☐
	b)	☒	☐
	c)	☐	☒
	d)	☒	☐
	e)	☐	☒
9.	a)	☐	☒
	b)	☒	☐
	c)	☒	☐
	d)	☒	☐
	e)	☐	☒
10.	a)	☐	☒
	b)	☐	☒
	c)	☒	☐
	d)	☐	☒
	e)	☐	☒
11.	a)	☐	☒
	b)	☒	☐
	c)	☒	☐
	d)	☐	☒
	e)	☒	☐
12.	a)	☒	☐
	b)	☐	☒
	c)	☒	☐
	d)	☐	☒
	e)	☒	☐
13.	a)	☐	☒
	b)	☒	☐
	c)	☒	☐
	d)	☐	☒
	e)	☒	☐
14.	a)	☐	☒
	b)	☒	☐
	c)	☒	☐
	d)	☒	☐
	e)	☐	☒
15.	a)	☒	☐
	b)	☐	☒
	c)	☒	☐
	d)	☒	☐
	e)	☐	☒
16.	a)	☐	☒
	b)	☒	☐
	c)	☐	☒
	d)	☐	☒
	e)	☐	☒
17.	a)	☐	☒
	b)	☒	☐
	c)	☒	☐
	d)	☐	☒
	e)	☐	☒
18.	a)	☐	☒
	b)	☐	☒
	c)	☐	☒
	d)	☒	☐
	e)	☒	☐
19.	a)	☒	☐
	b)	☒	☐
	c)	☐	☒
	d)	☒	☐
	e)	☒	☐
20.	a)	☒	☐
	b)	☒	☐
	c)	☐	☒
	d)	☐	☒
	e)	☒	☐

Index

Teachers' Guide

Teaching First Aid

First Aid Step by Step is the first book of its kind aimed specially at young readers. The object is to teach teenagers the principles of First Aid so that when a crisis arises now, or later in adult life, they will be able to deal with it in an intelligent and knowledgeable way.
The modern school curriculum includes topics of practical value to the student in his school career and throughout his life. Some subjects have become obsolete in the secondary school, and new topics such as home economics, human biology and first aid have been introduced as an integral part of the curriculum. Until now no text specifically for teaching First Aid has been available. *First Aid Step by Step* fulfils this need. In its 128 pages, the student will find practical solutions to all basic first aid emergencies, their medical background and 150 precise drawings to illustrate the text. First Aid is not a subject to be learnt for examinations and then promptly forgotten; it is a practical skill which enables the first aider to act intelligently and calmly in an emergency. The first person to arrive at an accident must be able to take charge and make the correct decisions if he is to save life, end suffering and help recovery. *First Aid Step by Step* is designed to help you teach this. It is up to the teacher to supplement the text in several ways:

(1) By demonstrating practical points such as the making of a ring bandage or a sling (there are teaching aids available to help you,—see Page 9).
(2) By stressing the correct order of priorities, viz; breathing, bleeding and care of the unconscious and making sure that the first aider gets first things first.
(3) By ensuring that the injured are treated gently. As you know, rough handling may produce further injury. If the victim is frightened and in pain, the first aider must realise that he is dealing with a physically and mentally distressed person.

It is important that teachers point out the difference between an uninjured volunteer who is being used to demonstrate a wound in the classroom, and a real, suffering casualty.

Organising the Course

Many examination syllabuses now contain elements of first aid, usually arterial bleeding, mouth to mouth resuscitation, shock and unconsciousness. Naturally, your course organisation may need to be tailored to meet the demands of one such syllabus. *First Aid Step by Step* is a comprehensive text which may contain subjects beyond your particular syllabus. In this case, select individual chapters relevant to your course.

Each chapter stands on its own, opening with an anecdote which presents with a life-threatening situation (e.g. Chapter 7, If Breathing Stops, begins with a drowning victim and asks the question 'what would you do to save his life?').

Then follows a section on the anatomy and physiology relevant to the problem, (e.g. in Chapter 7, the process of breathing and the causes of failure to breath are explained and illustrated in this section). Next comes Step by Step in which the practical solution to the problem is given. The chapter is completed by a quiz which highlights its main points.

First Aid Step by Step, can be altered to fit any particular course. If there is little time available the theory section may be omitted, going straight from the opening anecdote to the step by step section. If your syllabus allows a generous amount of time for first aid, work thoroughly through the book and include some of the projects and audiovisual aids given on pages 9-10 of this section.

1 Is it a poison?

The overdose has reached epidemic proportions. The incidence of addiction to dangerous drugs and to alcohol is rising rapidly and is now a serious problem, particularly in the teenage group. This chapter explains the emergency treatment of acute poisoning, stressing as a priority the prevention of such emergencies. In the overdose situation, poisons are divided into two groups: corosive and non-corosive,—an important distinction because of their different treatments. Accidental poisoning from garden plants, chemicals, stings and bites are reviewed. Specific antedotes to poisons are not important to the first aider, but their general treatment and their prevention are particularly relevant to the age group most vulnerable to this problem. The treatment and prevention of addiction to dangerous drugs, although not previously included in the repertoire of the First Aider, must now be considered the responsibility of all.

2 Coping with a burn

The structure and function of the skin and the problems produced by skin loss due to burns is the content of the theory section in this chapter. The treatment of burns should stress prevention of further damage: by cooling to reduce retained heat, by removing constrictions such as rings to prevent loss of blood supply, by dressing to prevent infection and by elevating and immobilising a burnt limb to prevent swelling.

Electrical and corrosive burns should be considered as special cases only in so far as the first aider needs to protect himself from suffering similar burns.

3 Out of joint

Soft tissue injuries such as sprains and dislocations are common on the sports-field and this chapter can be thought of as a compendium of common sporting injuries. Although distinctions are made between the various forms of injury their treatments are the same. Cold water, compression and elevation of the injured part, is the usual treatment for any of these injuries. The old-fashioned sponge of cold water or the modern cold aerosol spray is the secret of the football trainer or efficient First Aider.

4 If a bone breaks

Bones are of different shapes and sizes and it is the long, thin bones of the limbs that are most frequently broken. Although the theory section of this chapter details the various functions of bone and the particular types of fracture, the most important section outlines the general treatment of a broken bone, e.g. immobilisation. The specific way in which fractures may be immobilised is contained in Appendix 2. Dealing with a particular fracture requires practical skill, patience and gentleness which can only be taught by a teacher.
When such a fracture has been immobilised, the casualty often needs transporting from the scene of the accident. Transport methods are illustrated in Appendix 3.

5 It's a knockout

The general treatment of the unconscious victim is straightforward—the casualty should be placed in the recovery or coma position. When this has been accomplished the First Aider should try to reach a diagnosis by examining the casualty, talking to witnesses and searching for clues such as Medic-Alert discs or bracelets. Coma may result from failure to breath, cardiac arrest or shock following excessive blood loss. In these cases, the casualty cannot be left in the recovery position; immediate treatment should begin to restore these vital functions. Once this is done the victim may then be placed in the recovery position.

You should stress that the unconscious casualty should be seen by a doctor irrespective of whether he regains consciousness. Epilepsy is an exception to this rule—unless the casualty has injured himself or has been unconscious for a prolonged period.

6 How to survive

This chapter focuses the attention on the problems of exposure to different climatic conditions. It is particularly relevent to school expeditions and field-studies. Again, prevention in the form of good planning is an important feature. It is necessary that the First Aider grasps the essential difference between cold exhaustion which attacks the ill-equipped mountaineer quickly reducing his body temperature, and severe hypothermia which is a condition in which the body is cooled slowly and drastically. In cold exhaustion the body should be heated quickly while in severe hypothermia rapid re-warming draws blood from vital organs and could kill.

7 If breathing stops

The opening anecdote in this chapter illustrates one common way in which breathing fails, i.e. drowning. Instruction in the technique of life saving in this situation includes the mouth to mouth method of artificial respiration. Younger children may find this process embarrassing, perhaps even frightening, and the teacher must help them to overcome their fears. In *First Aid Step by Step* older methods of artificial ventilation such as the Holger-Neilson or Sylvester techniques have not been discussed because they are by no means as efficient or reliable as the exhaled air method. There are, however, occasional situations where these other mechanisms of assisted ventilation are useful, e.g. when the mouth or pharynx is burnt or physically inaccessible. You may wish to teach your students these methods as an alternative to the mouth to mouth technique.
Artificial ventilation and maintenance of an airway represents one of the most useful forms of First Aid assistance. Many lives may be saved by prompt attention to breathing faults.

8 How to control bleeding

This is a large and important chapter. It not only explains internal and external bleeding but covers the state of shock. The treatment of external bleeding is a priority in First Aid. Many victims of road accidents, for example, die simply because bleeding is not controlled. The sight of blood frightens many people and the teacher must try to get his First Aiders used to seeing blood by simulating it in the classroom. It should be realised that a little blood may look much more than its actual volume.
The official First Aid organisations have in recent years tried to discourage the use of tourniquets which if applied for too long a period may result in the loss of a limb through gangrene. Instead direct pressure on arterial pressure points is recommended. These points are illustrated and explained in the text but each student should be made familiar with their location by feeling for their own arterial pulses.
Because of the importance of this topic it may well be sensible to spend several sessions on it. If this is not possible concentrate on:
(1) The treatment of external bleeding.
(2) The recognition and treatment of shock.

9 When the heart stops

In this section is described a method of supporting the circulation by physically compressing the heart between the breast bone and the back bone to eject blood into the circulation. It is important that the student has an opportunity to try this method but he should not, of course, practise on his friends because it is both painful and dangerous. There are a variety of dummies commercially available. If the school funds do not allow the purchase of one of these it would be an easy and interesting project for the class to construct a suitable model on which to practise.
In reality when the heart stops breathing rapidly fails and both external cardiac compression and artificial ventilation must be performed at the same time. Several schemes for doing both procedures are recommended in chapter 9. It is therefore preferable to cover assisted ventilation before considering cardiac resuscitation. Now that it is possible for First Aiders to artificially maintain the circulation and ventilation it must be understood that the unfortunate victim is not dead until the First Aider stops or is unable to continue this artificial support.

10 Just an ache or pain

Aches and pains are common complaints often not of a serious nature. A simple remedy may be available but if not a mild pain-killing drug can be advised. Until recently aspirin preparations were recommended but the official First Aid organisations now suggest that paracetamol is a safer alternative. Of course, any pain which does not respond to these simple measures should be referred to a doctor. On no account should a dose of one paracetamol tablet every two hours be exceeded. If the pain continues First Aiders must advise the victim to seek a doctor's opinion.

11 Dealing with disaster

Road traffic accidents and other disasters are part of modern life. Everyone will on average at some time in his life be a witness to a major accident. Here every variety of injury will be found. In this situation a First Aider will be of great value to the injured victims if he remains level headed and remembers his basic First Aid. It is often difficult to keep calm and because of this Chapter 11 contains precise instructions on how to act. Safety first and the correct order of First Aid treatment are the most important points to remember. Classroom simulation of an accident situation will help to reinforce the correct steps to take in an emergency.
Dealing with disaster also includes advice on how to cope with the variety of human reactions likely to be found at an accident.

The Appendices

The application of bandages and dressings (Appendix 1), the immobilisation of specific fractures (Appendix 2), and the transportation of injured casualties (Appendix 3) are all described diagrammatically in the appendices. This information has been removed from the text where it usually obscures the important general points of treatment. The techniques which are illustrated require personal demonstration by an instructor and repeated practice by the First Aider.
Appendix 4 is a compendium of technical terms used by First Aiders. Many other words could be included but the over use of technical terminology is not necessary.

Quizzes and Final Test

Questions have been included simply to evaluate the student's grasp of basic first aid.

First Aid is a practical skill best learned by constant practice. As in other subjects imaginative projects improve the quality of both teaching and learning. Here are some you may want to try with your students:

Casualty simulation

With the help of greasepaint, powder and plasticine it is possible to recreate many lifelike first aid situations—arms may be 'burnt', limbs 'broken' and casualties 'shocked' etc. But some features, such as a fast heart rate or a bleeding artery, cannot be easily or safely reproduced. Enthusiasts have developed techniques for imitating severed arteries with rubber tubing and pumps. This particular scheme can be used to show children how much pressure is required to stop a bleeding artery or vein.

It is safe for children to practise mouth to mouth respiration on each other. If this is done under supervision in the classroom they will know how to act in an emergency. Do not let them try external cardiac compression as it can be dangerous. Adequate practice in this technique must be achieved by using a specially designed model such as Rescuci Anne or a similar classroom-built model.

Making first aid slides

A whole and complete variety of illustrated slides may be bought or hired from educational suppliers but this may prove expensive. It is quite easy to make your own set of colour slides using simulated victims and step by step treatment. 8 mm films and 35 mm filmstrips are available from the first aid organisations, health education authorities, drug companies and medical charities. Posters and wall charts may be purchased but can also be produced as class projects.

Competitions

Official First Aid organisations, industrial First Aid groups, mountain rescue teams and other life-saving groups often organise competitions

to stimulate and maintain interest in the five points of First Aid. These competitions usually call for a simple injury to be treated by one person or a more complex situation by a team of First Aiders under the watchful eyes of trained medical or first aid personnel. The tests are easy to design, simple to mark and enjoyable to perform.
Tests should emphasise the following features:

Correct assessment of priorities.
Rapid and efficient application of First Aid.
Improvisation of equipment.
Proper safety precautions.
Arrangements for casualty disposal.

Training of first aid teams

It should be possible to train children adequately to form a squad of student First Aiders who could be asked to be on duty at appropriate school occasions e.g. Sports Days and Saturday sporting events.

Visiting hospitals and medical schools

Professional First Aiders, doctors and nurses are usually very helpful to young and enthusiastic First Aiders. Visits to the local ambulance station, fire station, St. John or Red Cross brigade, or hospital can be arranged. Representatives from these units are often willing to make occasional school visits to instruct the children.

First aid procedures

The treatment recommended in *First Aid Step By Step* conforms with the official procedures used by First Aid organisations

Fashion and future in first aid

Throughout *First Aid Step by Step* the advice given is similar to that of the official First Aid organizations. With every revision of First Aid textbooks new techniques are suggested and older methods rejected. Some of the old methods may be better than the new techniques.

Broken collar bone

The victim with a fractured clavicle usually sits supporting his arm to lessen the pain from the broken collar bone. It is good theoretical advice to place bandages around both shoulders and pull them back with a third bandage across the back. Real casualties often reject this treatment and simulated casualties have been known to faint when this treatment has been applied. The old treatment of a thick pad under the arm and a triangular sling is much better.

Saline emetics

One method of treating non-corrosive poisons is to induce vomiting. This can be achieved by getting the victim to take a tumbler of water in which two tablespoons of salt have been dissolved. It has been recognized for some time that repeated doses should not be given because of the danger of salt poisoning. However, several fatal cases of salt poisoning have resulted from one dose of the above prescription. These have usually occurred in children and we feel that the official recommendation should not include salt and water administration to poisoned children.

Burns, crash injury and shock

It is usually stated that a shocked casualty should be given nothing by mouth. Burns and crash injury both produce shock and yet in both cases modest quantities of water by mouth are recommended. This creates such confusion amongst First Aiders that we feel that no water should be given to victims of burns or crash injury.

Artificial ventilation

In the case of drowning, many teach the preliminary use of a mechanical method of artificial ventilation. This wastes time and is a relatively inefficient method. Whenever possible the exhaled air method (mouth to mouth/nose) should be started immediately.

Cardiac resuscitation

There is a great deal of argument and disagreement about the technique of cardiac resuscitation. The present advice of ten sharp blows to the sternum followed by external cardiac compression is difficult to understand and far from logical. Children should be taught only the simple technique of external cardiac compression. Adults could adopt a more rational approach: one heavy blow with the edge of a closed fist to the lower half of the breastbone may shock an electrically disorganized (ventricular fibrulation) heart into good electrical order. If a continued cardia action follows this treatment then no other cardia resuscitation is necessary. If no pulse follows this blow then external cardiac compression should be started immediately without wasting time by striking the chest again. If the blow is accompanied by one pulse only the First Aider should try simply tapping on the breast bone – in a small proportion of cases this may result in a pulse each time the breast-bone is tapped. This may be sufficient to sustain life. If there is no pulse when the breastbone is tapped then external cardiac compression is necessary.

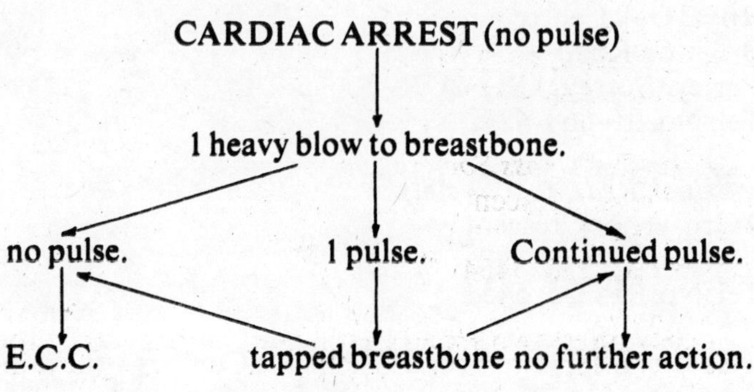

Useful addresses and First Aid courses

(1) *British Association of Sport and Medicine*
Hon. Secretary: Dr P. N. Serryn
63 Alric Avenue
New Malden, Surrey
Tel. No: 01-949 0607

(2) *The Duke of Edinburgh Award*
Head Office: 2 Old Queen Street
Westminster
London SW1H 9HR
Tel. No: 01–930 7681

There are also offices in Wallsend; Abbots Bromley, Dr Rugeley; Burscough, near Ormskirk; Milton Keynes; Bromley; Taunton; Cardiff; Edinburgh and Belfast. Addresses are available from Head Office. About 100,000 young people take part in the scheme through schools and First Aid is a popular choice. The instruction is tied to the Certificate Examinations of the Red Cross and St. John Ambulance Brigade and both instruction and assessment are carried out by their officers. Contact one of the Duke of Edinburgh Award offices for full details.

(3) *The Medical Committee on Accident Prevention*
50 Old Brompton Road
London, SW7 3EA
Tel. No: 01–584 9240

(4) *The Royal Society for the Prevention of Accidents (ROSPA)*
Royal Oak Centre
Brighton Road
Purley, Surrey, CR2 2UR
Tel. No: 01–668 4272

(5) *The British Red Cross Society*
9 Grosvenor Crescent
London SW1
Tel. No: 01–235 5454

The Society offers two broad Certificate Courses—the junior and

the senior. The junior category is normally taken by those young people who are studying for the bronze award in the Duke of Edinburgh Award Scheme. It is also possible for schools to use this course.
In the senior category the most popular course is the Adult Initial. This is the course used for industry and successful candidates are issued a certificate which is recognised by various Government Ministries.

(6) *The St. John Ambulance Brigade*
1 Grosvenor Cresent
London SW1X 7EF
Tel. No: 01–235 5231

The Brigade runs various certificate courses. *Essentials of First Aid* is open to the 11–16 age group and is the one used in the bronze and silver Dukc of Edinburgh Award schemes The *Standard First Aid* course is for 16 year olds and over and is used in the gold Duke of Edinburgh Awards.

(7) *The St. Andrew Brigade*
The St. Andrew Brigade covers Scotland and offers the same courses as the St. John Brigade.

Further reading

Anatomy and Physiology

Illustrated Physiology. McNaught and Callander (Churchill Livingstone).
Companion to Illustrated Physiology, McNaught and Callander (Churchill Livingstone).
Anatomy and Physiology for Nurses, Sears (Edward Arnold).

Dictionaries

Nurses Dictionary, (Baillière, Tindall)
Fabers Nurses' Dictionary

Drugs and Alcohol

Face the Facts, The Rev. D. J. Tizzard, 'Elston', The Avenue, Truro, Cornwall.

First Aid

Baillière's: Handbook of First Aid, edited by Stanley Miles.
New Advanced First Aid, A. Ward Gardner and Peter J. Roylance (Butterworths).
First Aid, The authorised Manual of St. John Ambulance Association and Brigade.

Teaching First Aid

Baillière's Teaching First Aid, Stanley Miles and Peter J. Roylance.
First Aid Questions and Answers, Compiled from The Authorised First Aid Manual of St. John Ambulance, St. Andrew's Ambulance Association, and The British Red Cross Society.

Rescue

Mountain Rescue, (HMSO)
Safety Afloat N. Zantvoort (Hollis and Carter)
Medical Care for Mountain Climbers, Steele (William Heinemann Medical Books)